In two successive years of the seventeenth century London suffered two terrible disasters. Throughout the spring and summer of 1665 an outbreak of bubonic plague spread among its inhabitants, striking parish after parish, until thousands had died and the huge pits dug to receive their bodies were full. At last it slowly declined, but in September of the next year a raging fire burned in the City, destroying countless houses and many famous buildings.

This book tells the story of these two tragic events by means of extracts from the writings of Londoners who were there at the time. These include Samuel Pepys and John Evelyn, the two diarists of the time, the Earl of Clarendon and Bishop Burnet, both important men in the state, clergymen and doctors who remained in town during both disasters, and Daniel Defoe, who was only a child during the Plague, but wrote an account of it based on the stories of those who had lived through those days. The book concludes with eyewitness accounts about the rebuilding of the ruined City, which transformed it at last from a medieval to a modern town.

Illustrated throughout with pictures drawn from contemporary sources, this addition to the WAYLAND DOCUMENTARY HISTORY SERIES, offers an exciting and authentic approach to history studies.

Frontispiece A contemporary view of the Great Fire of London 1666

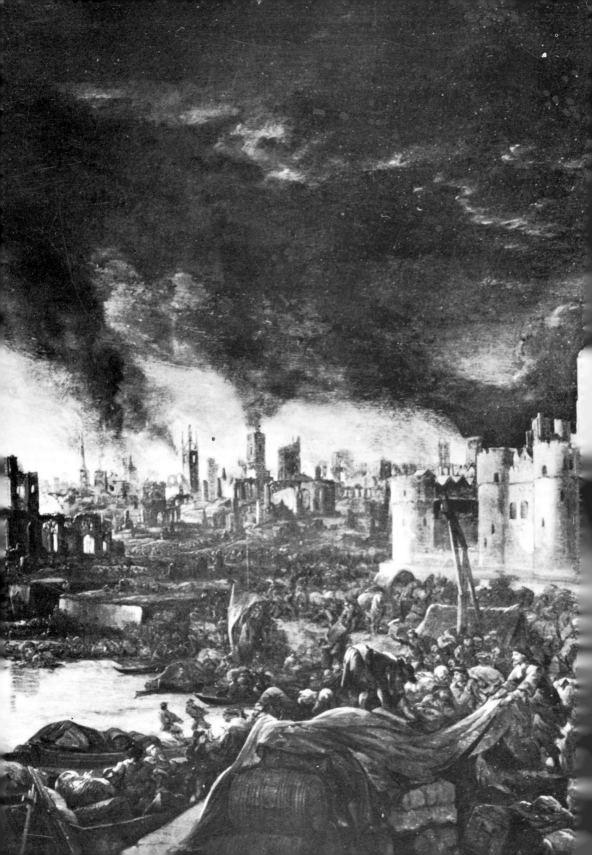

Plague and Fire

London 1665–66

by Leonard W. Cowie

WAYLAND PUBLISHERS

SBN (hardback edition): 85340 007 5
Fourth impression 1977
Copyright © 1970 by Wayland (Publishers) Ltd
49 Lansdowne Place, Hove, East Sussex BN3 1HF
Photoset by BAS Printers Limited, Wallop, Hampshire
Printed by Clarke, Doble & Brendon Ltd
Plymouth and London

Contents

The Illustrations

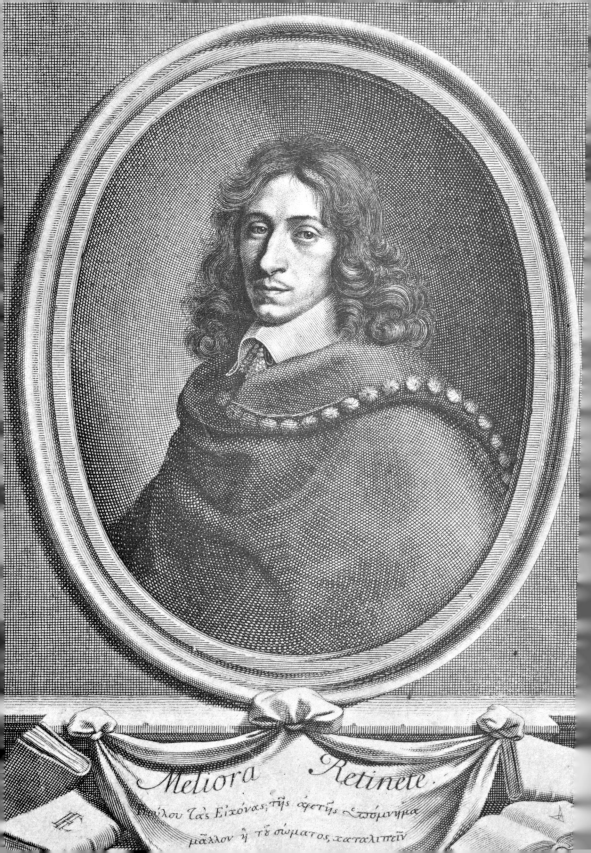

Meliora Retinete.

Παύλου τὰς Εἰχόνας, τῆς ἀρετῆς ὑπόμνημα
μᾶλλον ἢ τῦ σώματος, χαταλιπεῖν

1 The Fearful City

FEW CHILDREN, when they dance to this nursery-rhyme (1), realize
that it goes back to the Great Plague in London; but a rosy rash
was a sign of the plague, posies of herbs were carried as a pro-
tection against it, sneezing was a common indication of approach-
ing death, and 'all fall down' was exactly what happened.

> Ring a-ring a-Roses
> A pocketful of posies,
> 'Tishoo, 'tishoo,
> We all fall down!

Seventeenth-century London had a population of 460,000
packed into decaying, wooden houses and narrow streets. John
Graunt, a Fellow of the Royal Society, wrote: 'London, the
Metropolis of England, is perhaps a Head too big for the Body ...
Our parishes are now grown madly disproportionable ... The old
streets are unfit for the present frequency of coaches (2).'

Since all the houses had coal fires, it was also a smoky, dirty
city. John Evelyn wrote in 1661 in a pamphlet: 'This horrid smoke
obscures our churches and makes our palaces look old. It fouls
our clothes and corrupts the waters, so that the very rain and
refreshing dews that fall in the several seasons precipitate this
impure vapour, which with its black and tenacious quality, spots
and contaminates whatever is exposed to it (3).'

Evelyn summed up his condemnation of the old City: 'That this
Glorious and Antient City ... should wrap her stately head in
Clowds of Smoake and Sulphur, so full of stink and Darknesse,
I deplore with just Indignation. That the Buildings should be

11

Facing page The diarist, John Evelyn (1620-1706)

composed of such a Congestion of mishapen and extravagant Houses; that the Streets should be so narrow and incommodious in the very Centre, and busiest places of Intercourse; That there should be so ill and uneasie a form of Paving under foot, so troublesome and malicious a disposure of the Spouts and Gutters overhead, are particular worthy of Reproof and Reformation; because it is hereby rendered a Labyrinth in its principal passages, and a continual wet day after the storm is over (4).'

Attempts to limit its size As early as Elizabeth I's reign, a Royal Proclamation had tried to prevent the growth of London's outskirts. It gave as the reason: 'The Queen's Majesty perceiving the state of the City of London and the suburbs and confines thereof to increase daily by access of people to inhabit the same ... and there are such great multitudes of people brought to inhabit in small rooms, whereof a great part are seen to be very poor; yea such must live of begging, or of worse means; and they heaped up together, and in a sort smothered with many families of children and servants in one house or small tenement; it must needs follow, if any plague or popular sickness should by God's permission enter among those multitudes, that the same should not only spread itself and invade the whole city and confines, as great mortality should ensue the same, but would be also dispersed through ... the realm (5).'

Past plagues This extract from *A Dialogue against the Pestilence* (1564) written by William Bullein is a reminder that for centuries London had suffered from visitations of plague:

Civis: Good wife, the daily jangling and ringing of the bells, the coming in of the Minister to every house in ministring the communion, in reading the homily of death, the digging up of graves, the sparring in of windows, and the blazing forth of the blue cross, do make my heart tremble and quake. Alas, what shall I do to save my life?

Uxor: Sir, we are but young, and have but a time in this world, what doth it profit us to gather riches together, and can not enjoy them? Why tarry we here so long? I do think every hour a year until we be gone ... seeing that we have sent our children forth three weeks past into a good air and a sweet country, let us follow them ... Let us take leave of our neighbours, and return merely home again when the plague is past, and the dog days ended. (6).'

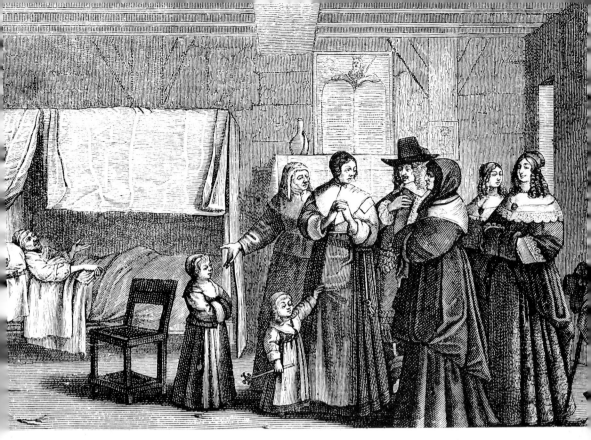

A doctor visiting the sick

Many Londoners feared that disaster would strike their city. *Plague and*
A clergyman, Thomas Reeve, wrote a pamphlet in 1657 in which *fire foretold*
he foretold the Plague: 'What inventions shall ye then be put
to … when your sins shall have shut up all the conduits of the city,
when ye shall see no men of your incorporation, but the mangled
citizen; nor hear no noise in your streets but the crys, the shrieks,
the yells and pangs of gasping, dying men; when among the
throngs of associates not a man will own you or come near
you? (7)'

Soon afterwards Thomas Reeve preached a sermon forecasting
the Fire: 'Can sin and the City's safety, can impenitence and
impurity stand long together? Fear you not some plague, some
coal blown with the breath of the Almighty, that may sparkle
and kindle, and burn you to such cinders that not a wall or pillar
may be left to testify the remembrance of the City? (8)'

13

A Quaker, Humphrey Smith, published a pamphlet called *A Vision*, which contained a description of London burning down: 'And the fire continued, for, though all the lofty part was brought down, yet there was much old stuffe, and parts of broken down desolate walls, which the fire continued burning against ... And the Vision thereof remained in me as a thing that was showed me of the Lord (9).'

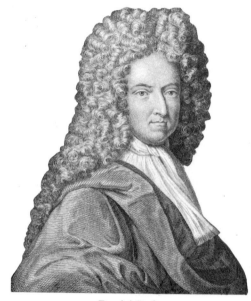

Daniel Defoe

Daniel Defoe was only five when the Plague came to London, but he later made use of memories and interviews to write a realistic account of the times. Here he describes how people believed that comets foretold both disasters: 'In the first place, a blazing star or comet appeared for several months before the plague, as there did the year after another, a little before the fire. The old women and the phlegmatic hypochondriac part of the other sex, whom I could almost call old women too, remarked (especially afterwards, though not till both those judgments were over) that those two comets passed directly over the city, and that so very near the houses that it was plain they imported something peculiar to the city alone; that the comet before the pestilence

14

was of a faint, dull, languid colour, and its motion very heavy, solemn, and slow; but that the comet before the fire was bright and sparkling, or, as others said, flaming, and its motion swift and furious; and that accordingly one foretold a heavy judgment, slow but severe, terrible and frightful, as was the plague; but the other foretold a stroke, sudden, swift, and fiery as the conflagration. Nay, so particular some people were, that as they looked upon that comet preceding the fire, they fancied that they not

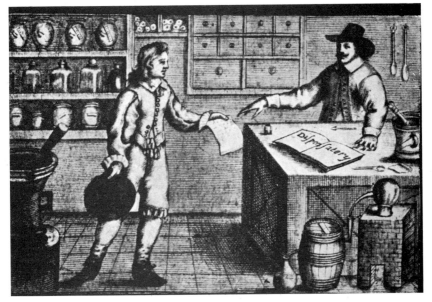

Dispensing a prescription in the seventeenth century

only saw it pass swiftly and fiercely, and could perceive the motion with their eye, but even they heard it; that it made a rushing, mighty noise, fierce, and terrible, though at a distance, and but just perceivable (10).'

Dr George Thomson, a London physician, supported the popular belief that the stars foretold disaster: 'That Comets, or Blazing Stars, do portend some Evil to come upon Mortals, is confirmed by long observation and sad experience, as likewise Phenomena of ... new Stars, Battles Fought and Coffins carried through the Air, Howlings, Screechings and Groans heard about Churchyards, also raining of Blood (11).'

A doctor's opinion

15

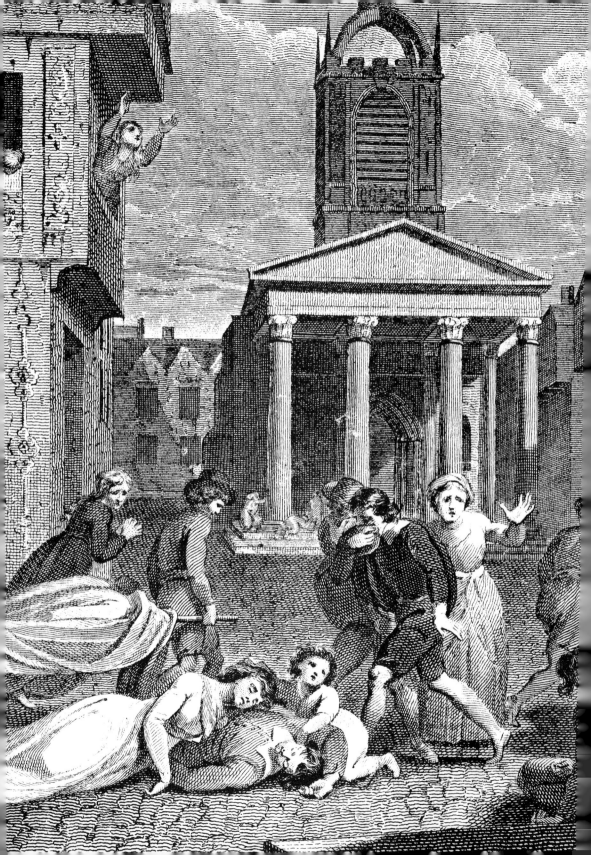

2 The Coming of the Plague

Plague appears

WHEN the Plague began in the bitter winter of 1664–5, England was at war with Holland. The Earl of Clarendon, then Lord Chancellor, told how people at first thought little of it and laughed at those who were worried: 'There begun now to appear another enemy, much more formidable than the Dutch, and more difficult to be struggled with; which was the plague, that brake out in the winter, and made such an early progress in the spring, that though the weekly numbers did not rise high, and it appeared to be only in the outskirts of the town, and in the most obscure alleys, amongst the poorest people; yet the ancient men, who well remembered in what manner the last great plague (which had been near forty years before) first brake out, and the progress it afterwards made, foretold a terrible summer. And many of them removed their families out of the city to country habitations; when their neighbours laughed at their providence, and thought they might have stayed without danger: but they found shortly that they had done wisely (12).'

A joke?

Sir Ralph Verney, up from the country, at first noted the outbreak in a letter merely in joke: 'Tis plaguey newes that the plague has come to Southwark (13).'

The Plague began in the poor, overcrowded parish of St Giles-in-the-Fields. Sir Thomas Peyton wrote bitterly afterwards: 'That one parish of St Giles at London hath done us all this mischief (14).'

Red crosses

Dr Thomas Vincent, a clergyman who stayed in London all the time, described how as the Plague spread, the victims and their families were kept in their houses and an ominous warning sign

17

Facing page A scene from the Great Plague

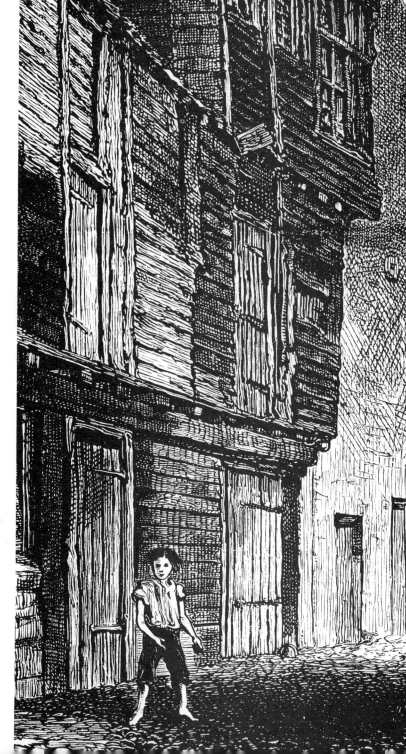

The first house
smitten by the
Plague, Ashlin's
Place, Drury Lane
in London

painted on the doors: 'It was very Dismal to behold the Red Crosses, and read in great letters "Lord Have Mercy Upon Us" on the doors, and Watchmen standing beside them with Halberts, and such a solitude about those places, and people passing by them so gingerly and with such fearful looks, as if they had been lined with enemies in ambush that waited to destroy them (15).'

Old women worked as 'searchers of the dead' to report deaths to the parish clerks, and the figures were published in the weekly *Bills of Mortality*: 'When any one dieth, either the Tolling or Ringing of the Bell, or the bespeaking of a Grave, intimateth to the Searchers (who keep a strict Correspondence with the Sexton), and thereupon the Ancient Matrons sworn to that Office, repair to the Place where the dead Corps lieth, and upon their own View, and others' Examination, make a Judgment by what Disease or Casualty the Corps died; which Judgment they report to the Parish Clerk (16).'

Bills of Mortality

Here is an example of an advertisement by a quack doctor early in 1665. Though he claimed to advise the poor for nothing, they found that he charged for the medicine he said would protect them from the Plague: 'An experienced Physician, who has long studied the doctrine of antidotes against all sorts of poison and infection, has, after forty years' practice, arrived to such skill as may, with God's blessing, direct persons how to prevent their being touched by any contagious distemper whatsoever. He directs the poor gratis (17).'

Quacks and Charms

The word Abracadabra, arranged in a triangle, was often found on charms which people bought from pedlars and wore to protect them against the Plague (18):

ABRACADABRA
ABRACADABR
ABRACADAB
ABRACADA
ABRACAD
ABRACA
ABRAC
ABRA
ABR
AB
A

Early in 1665, as Clarendon recalled, the Plague showed signs of abating: 'After Christmas the rage and fury of the pestilence began in some degree to be mitigated, but so little, that nobody who had left the town had yet the courage to return thither: nor had they reason; for though it was a considerable abatement from the height it had been at, yet there died still between three and four thousand in the week, and of those, some men of better condition than had fallen before (19).'

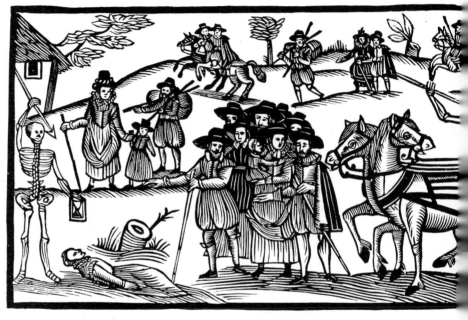

Townspeople fleeing into the countryside from an earlier plague

The King and the plague

Charles II was at Oxford, but as the Plague seemed to be slackening, his advisers thought he should come nearer to London. The 'general' mentioned by Clarendon was George Monk, Duke of Albemarle, Governor of the City: 'Windsor was thought upon as a place where the king might safely reside, there being then no infection there: but the king had adjourned the term thither, which had possessed the whole town; and he was not without some apprehension, that the plague had got into one house.

'In the end, towards the end of February, the king resolved that the queen and duchess and all their families should remain in Oxford; and that his majesty and his brother, with prince Rupert, and such of his council and other servants as were thought necessary or fit, would make a quick journey to Hampton-Court, where the general might be every day, and return again to London at night, and his majesty gave such orders as were requisite for the carrying on his service, and so after two or three days' stay there

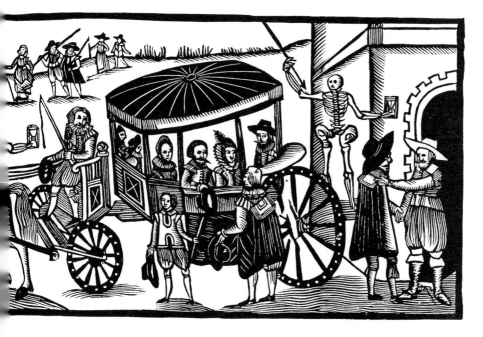

return again to Oxford; for no man did believe it counsellable, that his majesty should reside longer there, than the despatch of the most important business required: and with this resolution his majesty made his journey to Hampton-Court (20).'

Clarendon thought the continued decline of the Plague was due to the very cold weather: 'It pleased God, that the next week after his majesty came thither, the number of those who died of the plague in the city decreased one thousand; and there was a strange universal joy there for the king's being so near. The

A welcome frost

weather was as it could be wished, deep snow and terrible frost, which very probably stopped the spreading of the infection, though it might put an end to those who were already infected, as it did, for in a week or two the number of the dead was very little diminished (21).'

The King Charles II now thought it safe for his family and himself to
returns reside again in Whitehall Palace in London, and Clarendon described how this cheered people's spirits: 'And after a fortnight's

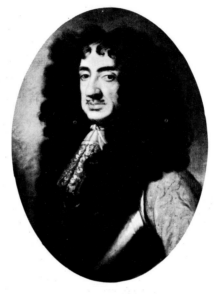

Charles II

or three weeks' stay, he resolved, for the quicker despatch of all that was to be done, to go to Whitehall, when there died above fifteen hundred in the week, and when there was not in a day seen a coach in the streets, but those which came in his majesty's train; so much all men were terrified from returning to a place of so much mortality. Yet it can hardly be imagined what numbers flocked thither from all parts upon the fame of the king's being at Whitehall, all men being ashamed of their fears for their own safety, when the king ventured his person. The judges at Windsor
22 adjourned the last return of the term to Westminster-hall, and

the town every day filled marvellously; and which was more wonderful, the plague every day decreased. Upon which the king changed his purpose, and, instead of returning to Oxford, sent for the queen and all the family to come to Whitehall (22).'

Nevertheless, Clarendon wrote, even when the King returned *False hopes* the Plague was getting worse with the warmer spring weather: 'So that before the end of March the streets were as full, the exchange as much crowded, and the people in all places as numer-

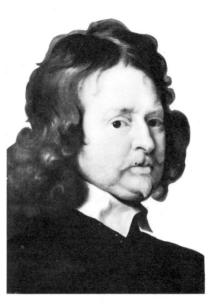

Edward Hyde, 1st Earl of Clarendon

ous, as they had ever been seen, few persons missing any of their acquaintance, though by the weekly bills there appeared to have died above one hundred and threescore thousand persons: and many, who could compute very well, concluded that there were in truth double that number who died; and that in one week, when the bill mentioned only six thousand, there had in truth fourteen thousand died (23).'

The revival of the Plague, Clarendon said, made Parliament *Parliament* decide to end its sittings, especially as many members had to take up war posts: 'In March it spread so much, that the parliament

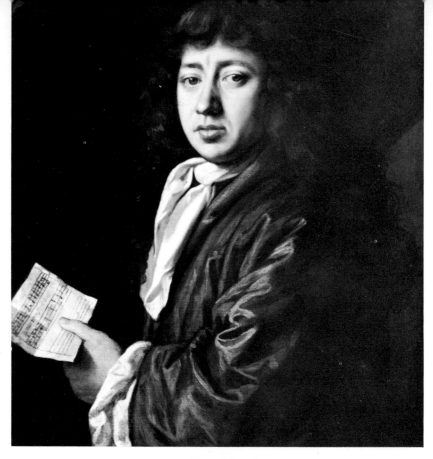

Samuel Pepys

was very willing to part: which was likewise the more necessary, in regard that so many of the members of the house of commons were assigned to so many offices and employments which related to the war, and which required their immediate attendance (24).'

On 30 April 1665 Samuel Pepys wrote fearfully in his diary about alarming talk he had heard in the City: 'Great fears of the sickenesse here in the City, it being said that two or three houses are already shut up. God preserve us all! (25).'

The Royalist journalist, Roger L'Estrange, who published the *Intelligencer*, tried to allay the alarm by pretending the plague was less serious in London than the King's Evil (scrofula). Early in May his newspaper announced: 'His Sacred Majesty, having declared it his Royal will and purpose to continue the healing of his people for the Evil during the month of May and then to give

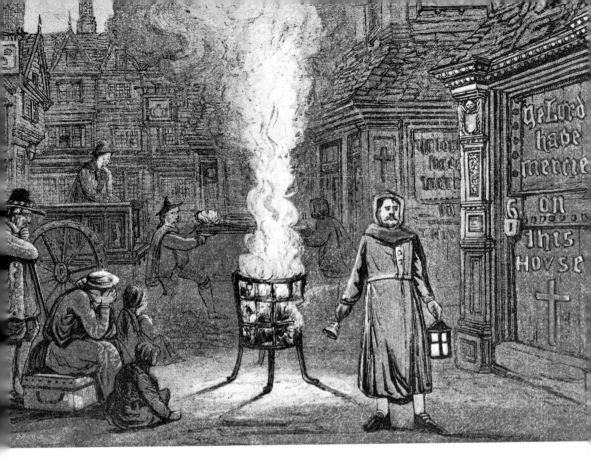

Watchmen in London during the Plague

over till Michaelmas next, I am commanded to give notice thereof that the people may not come up to Town in the Interim and lose their labour (26).'

But Defoe described the despair of people, who had trusted in the popular remedies, as the Plague spread: 'For when the plague evidently spread itself, they soon began to see the folly of trusting to those unperforming creatures who had gulled them of their money; and then their fears worked another way, namely to amazement and stupidity, not knowing what course to take or what to do either to help or relieve themselves. But they ran about from one neighbour's house to another, and even in the streets, from one door to another, with repeated cries of "Lord, have mercy upon us! What shall we do?" (27)'

In May Sir Ralph Verney wrote: ''Tis an ill time to put out

Growing alarm

25

money for the feare of the Plague makes many willing to take their Estates out of the Goldsmiths' hands, & the King's greate want of money makes many very unwilling to lend any money to these that advance greate summs for him (28).'

Death figures L'Estrange continued to try to allay alarm, and on 5 June his *Intelligencer* published figures of deaths from the Plague which were false, being probably only a third of the correct number: 'There are such Reports Spread abroad of the multitudes that dye weekly of the Plague in this Town, that for better information I shall briefly deliver the Truth of the matter. There have died three, and nine, and fourteen and seventeen in these four last weeks, forty-three in all, and none of these within the walls, and but five Parishes infected of 130 (29).'

Clarendon explained why even the official *Bills of Mortality* could not be accurate: 'The frequent deaths of the clerks and sextons of parishes hindered the exact account every week; but that which left it without any certainty was the vast number that was buried in the fields, of which no account was kept. Then of the anabaptists and other sectaries, who abounded in the city, very few left their habitations; and multitudes of them died, whereof no churchwarden or other officer had notice; but they found burials according to their own fancies, in small gardens or the next fields (30).'

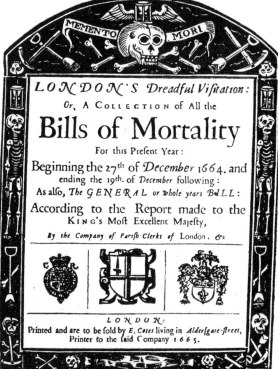

26

Title page of one of the *Bills of Mortality*

3 The Spread of Death and Fear

ON 7 JUNE Pepys saw the first signs of the Plague: 'This day, much *Pepys sees* against my will, I did in Drury Lane see two or three houses *the Plague* marked with a red cross upon the doors, and "Lord have Mercy upon us" writ there; which was a sad sight to me, being the first of the kind that, to my remembrance, I ever saw. It put me into an ill conception of myself and my smell, so that I was forced to buy some roll-tobacco to smell to and chaw, which took away the apprehension (31).'

On a hot afternoon in the middle of June Pepys took a coach ride which ended in this way: 'It struck me very deep this afternoon going with a hackney coach from my Lord Treasurer's down Holborne, the coachman I found to drive easily and easily, at last stood still, and come down hardly able to stand, and told me that he was suddenly struck very sicke, and almost blind, he could not see. So I 'light and went into another coach with a sad heart for the poor man and trouble for myself lest he should have been struck with the plague, being at the end of the towne that I took him up; but God have mercy upon us all! (32)'

The Plague now spread to the City itself. Defoe recounted what *Evacuation of* the wealthier people and the King and his court did: 'The city *London* itself began now to be visited too, I mean within the walls; but the number of people there were indeed extremely lessened by so great a multitude having been gone into the country; and even all this month of July they continued to flee, though not in such multitudes as formerly. In August, indeed, they fled in such a manner that I began to think there would be really none but magistrates and servants left in the city.

'As they fled now out of the city, so I should observe that the Court removed early, viz., in the month of June, and went to Oxford, where it pleased God to preserve them; and the distemper did not, as I heard of, so much as touch them, for which I cannot say that I ever saw they showed any great token of thankfulness, and hardly anything of reformation, though they did not want being told that their crying vices might, without breach of charity, be said to have gone far in bringing that terrible judgment upon the whole nation (33).'

Full coaches and waggons Pepys observed on 21 June: 'To the Cross Keys at Cripplegate, where I find all the towne almost going out of towne, the coaches and waggons being all full of people going into the country (34).'

The next day Pepys decided to send his mother into the country: 'In great pain whether to send my mother into the country to-day or no, I hearing that she, poor wretch, hath a mind to stay a little longer. At last I resolved to put it to her, and she agreed to go, so I would not oppose it, because of the sicknesse in the towne, and my intentions of removing my wife. So I did give her money and took a kind leave of her, and left my wife and people to see her out of town, and I at the office all the morning. At noon my wife tells me that she is with much ado gone, and I pray God bless her, but it seems she was to the last unwilling to go, but would not say so, but put it off till she lost her place in the coach, and was fain to ride in the waggon part (35).'

Pest houses The parish authorities set up improvised hospitals or 'pest-houses' for poor who caught the Plague. Here are extracts from parish accounts about the expenses incurred there (36):

Item given to severall poore people at the pest howse and to take away to [two] orphants from thence   .   .   .   .   .   . 10s.
To Anthony Halfield his children and hee being all sick [at margin, "dead."]   .   .   .   . 12s. 6d.
Item paid to John Alordin towards the buriall of his wiffe being poore and ded of the sickness and having 4 more in family   . . 11s.
Item paid to helpe buery John Alordin and his kinsman both of the visitation   .   .   .   . 2s.

Fear in the villages Often people who fled into the country found that the villages turned them away for fear of infection. Defoe recounted one such sad incident: 'There was one unhappy citizen, within my know-

28

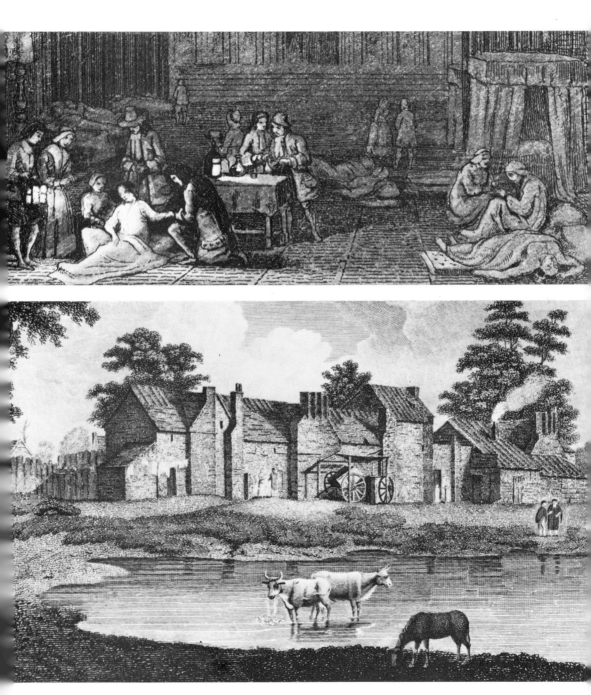

Top St Paul's Cathedral was converted into a pest-house during the
Bottom the pest-house in Tothill Fields outside London

ledge, who had been visited in a dreadful manner, so that his wife and all his children were dead, and himself and two servants only left, with an elderly woman, a near relation, who had nursed those that were dead as well as she could. This disconsolate man goes to a village near the town, though not within the bills of mortality, and finding an empty house there, inquires out the owner, and took the house. After a few days he got a cart and loaded it with goods, and carries them down to the house; the people of the village opposed his driving the cart along, but with some arguings and some force, the men that drove the cart along got through the street up to the door of the house. There the constable resisted them again, and would not let them be brought in. The man caused the goods to be unloaden and laid at the door, and sent the cart away; upon which they carried the man before a justice of peace; that is to say, they commanded him to go, which he did. The justice ordered him to cause the cart to fetch away the goods again, which he refused to do; upon which the justice ordered the constable to pursue the carters and fetch them back, and make them reload the goods and carry them away, or to set them in the stocks till they came for further orders; and if they could not find them, nor the man would not consent to take them away, they should cause them to be drawn with hooks from the house-door and burned in the street. The poor distressed man upon this fetched the goods again, but with grievous cries and lamentations at the hardship of his case. But there was no remedy; self-preservation obliged the people to those severities, which they would not otherwise have been concerned in (37).'

Escape up the river Defoe describes how the watermen, who ferried people in boats along the Thames, tried to escape with their families: 'Likewise I found that the watermen on the river above the bridge found means to convey themselves away up the river as far as they could go, and that they had, many of them, their whole families in their boats, covered with tilts and bales, as they call them and furnished with straw within for their lodging, and that they lay thus all along by the shore in the marshes, some of them setting up little tents with their sails, and so lying under them on shore in the day, and going into their boats at night; and in this manner, as I have heard, the river-sides were lined with boats and people as long as they had

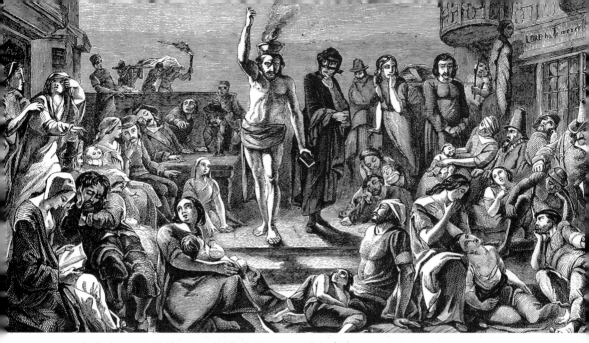

A madman, Solomon Eagle, preaching repentance during the Plague

anything to subsist on, or could get anything of the country (38).'

To Dr Vincent, the Plague was a just punishment for guilty sinners: 'The old drunkards, and swearers, and unclean persons, see many fellow-sinners fall before their faces, expecting every hour themselves to be smitten; and the very sinking fears they have of the Plague, hath brought the Plague and Death upon many; some by the sight of a Coffin in the Streets, have fallen into a shivering, and immediately the Disease hath assaulted them, and Serjeant Death hath arrested them (39).' *Punishment for sinners?*

Dr Thomas Gumble, the Duke of Albemarle's Chaplain, noticed, however, that the Plague struck indiscriminately: 'Death, as it were, rode triumphant through every street, as if it would have given no quarter to any of mankind, and ravaged as if it would have swallowed all mortality. It was a grievous sight to see in that great Emporie, nothing … merchantable but Coffins. (40).'

Richard Baxter, a Puritan minister, agreed with him: 'The richer sort removing out of the city, the greatest blow fell on the poor. At the first so few of the religiouser sort were taken away that (according to the mode of too many such) they began to be puffed up and boast of the great difference which God did make. But quickly after they all fell alike … (41).'

31

People were especially afraid of catching the Plague when buying food, and Defoe showed how they tried to avoid this: 'It is true people used all possible precaution. When any one bought a joint of meat in the market they would not take it off the butcher's hand, but took it off the hooks themselves. On the other hand, the butcher would not touch the money, but have it put into a pot full of vinegar, which he kept for that purpose. The buyer carried always small money to make up any odd sum, that they might take no change. They carried bottles of scents and perfumes in their hands, and all the means that could be used were used; but then the poor could not do even these things, and they went at all hazards (42).'

Defoe also recounted the elaborate precautions taken by an inn-keeper in picking up a lost purse, which might have belonged to someone who had caught the Plague: 'So he went in and fetched a pail of water, and set it down hard by the purse, then went again and fetched some gun-powder, and cast a good deal of powder upon the purse, and then made a train from that which he had thrown loose upon the purse. The train reached about two yards. After this he goes in a third time and fetches out a pair of tongs red hot, and which he had prepared, I suppose, on purpose, and first setting fire to the train of powder, that singed the purse, and also smoked the air sufficiently. But he was not content with that, but he then takes up the purse with the tongs, holding it so long till the tongs burnt through the purse, and then he shook the money out into the pail of water, so he carried it in. The money, as I remember, was about thirteen shillings and some smooth groats and brass farthings (43).'

Defoe noted the terror that possessed people in the worst-stricken area: 'One day, being at that part of the town on some special business, curiosity led me to observe things more than usually, and indeed I walked a great way where I had no business. I went up Holborn, and there the street was full of people, but they walked in the middle of the great street, neither on one side or other, because, as I suppose, they would not mingle with anybody that came out of houses, or meet with smells and scents from houses that might be infected (44).'

Pepys also observed the fear that was taking hold of people:

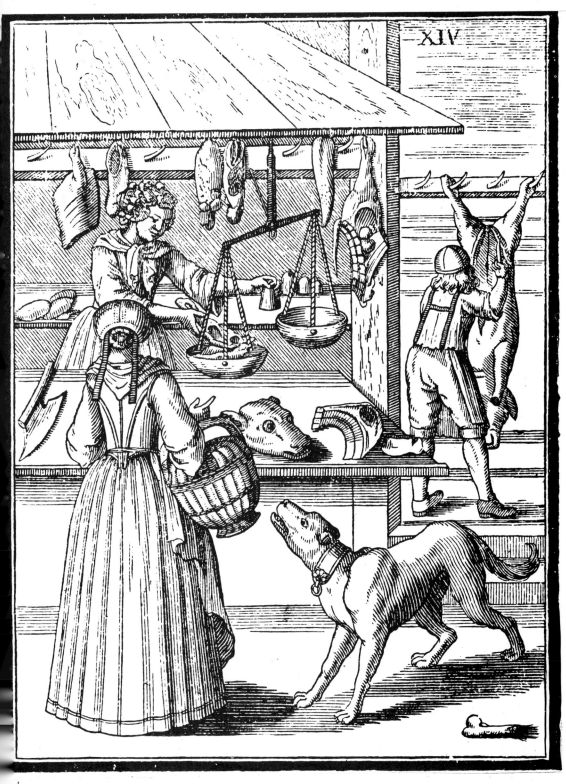

A butcher's shop about the time of the Great Plague

'Up, and being ready I out to the goldsmith's, having not for some days been in the streets; but now how few people I see, and those looking like people that had taken leave of the world (45).'

Vincent too was saddened at how empty and lonely London was in those days: 'Every day looks with the face of a Sabbath-day. Now shops are shut in, people rare and very few that walk about, insomuch that the grass begins to spring in some places, and a deep silence is almost every place, especially within the walls; no ratling Coaches, no prancing Horses, no calling in Customers, nor offering Wares, no London-Cryes sounding in the ears (46).'

An innkeeper announced his departure from London in the *Intelligencer*: 'This is to notify that the master of the Cock and Bottle, commonly called the Cock Alehouse, at Temple Bar, hath dismissed his servants, and shut up his house, for this long Vacation, intending (God willing) to return at Michaelmas next, so that all persons whatsoever who have any accompts with the said master, or farthings (tokens) belonging to the said house, are desired to repair thither before the 8th of this instant July, and they shall receive satisfaction (47).'

When houses were shut up because there had been a case of the Plague there, the people inside often tried to escape. They often killed the watchman stationed outside to keep them in. Defoe mentioned two such incidents: 'For example, in Coleman Street there are abundance of alleys, as appears still. A house was shut up in that they call White's Alley, and this house had a back-window, not a door, into a court, which had a passage into Bell Alley. A watchman was set by the constable, at the door of this house, and there he stood, or his comrade, night and day, while the family went all away in the evening out of that window into the court, and left the poor fellows warding ... for near a fortnight.

'Not far from the same place they blew up a watchman with gunpowder, and burned the poor fellow dreadfully; and while he made hideous cries, and nobody would venture to come near to help him, the whole family that were able to stir got out at the windows one storey high, two that were left sick calling out for help. Care was taken to give them nurses to look after them, but the persons fled were never found till after the plague was abated they returned; but as nothing could be proved, so nothing could be done to them (48).'

A contemporary writer tersely described the fate of those that remained confined in their houses: 'No drop of water, perhaps, but

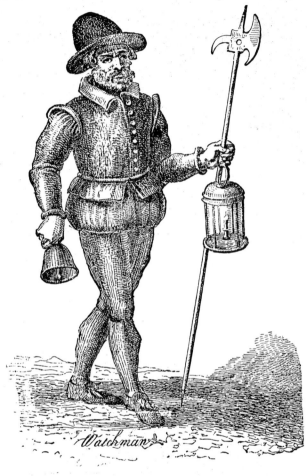

A London watchman at the time of the Plague

what comes at the leisure of a drunken or careless halberd bearer at the door; no seasonable provision is theirs as a certainty for their support. Not a friend to come nigh them in their many, many heart and house cares and complexities. They are compelled, though well, to lie by, to watch upon the death-bed of their dear relation, to see the corpse dragged away before their eyes. Affrighted children stand howling by their side. Thus they are fitted by fainting affliction to receive the impressions of a thousand fearful thoughts, in that long night they have to reckon with before release, as the family, so dismally exposed, sink one after another in the den of this dismal likeness of Hell, contrived by the advice of the English College of Doctors (49).'

Dr Hodges said that many Plague sufferers were more afraid of the nurses sent to look after them than of the Plague itself: 'But what greatly contributed to the loss of people thus shut up was the wicked practices of the nurses, for they are not to be mentioned but in the most bitter terms. These wretches, out of greediness to plunder the dead, would strangle their patients, and charge it to the distemper in their throats. Others would secretly convey the

The residence of the Lord Mayor of London in 1665

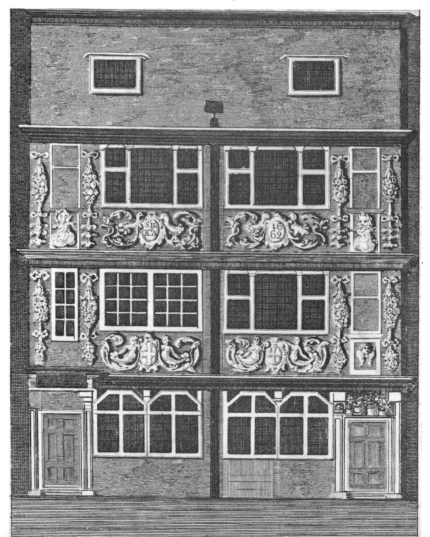

pestilential taint from sores of the infected to those who were well. Nothing, indeed, deterred these abandoned miscreants from prosecuting their avaricious purposes by all the methods their wickedness could invent. Although they were without witnesses to accuse them, yet it is not doubted but Divine Vengeance will overtake such wicked barbarities with due punishment. And so many were the artifices of these barbarous wretches, that it is to be hoped posterity will take warning how they trust them again in like cases (50).'

On 1 July, the Lord Mayor and Aldermen issued this order: 'It is thought necessary, and so ordered, that every householder do cause the street to be daily prepared before his door, and so to keep it clean swept all the week long (51).' *Emergency steps*

The Lord Mayor and Court of Aldermen at the time of the Plague

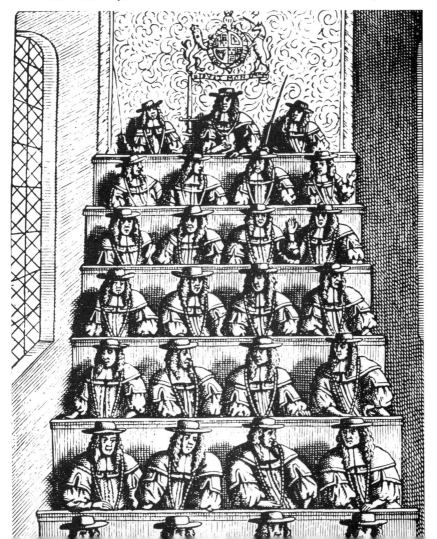

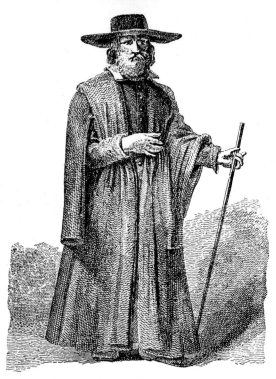

A corpse-bearer during the Plague

They also issued orders about the burial of those who had died
from the Plague: 'That the burial of the dead by this visitation be
at most convenient hours, always either before sun-rising or after
sun-setting, with the privity of the church-wardens or constable,
and not otherwise; and that no neighbours nor friends be suffered
to accompany the corpse to church, or to enter the house visited,
upon pain of having his house shut up or be imprisoned.

'And that no corpse dying of infection shall be buried, or remain
in any church in time of common prayer, sermon, or lecture. And
that no children be suffered at time of burial of any corpse in any
church, churchyard, or burying-place to come near the corpse,
coffin, or grave. And that all the graves shall be at least six feet
deep.

'And further, all public assemblies at other burials are to be for-
borne during the continuance of this visitation (52).'

Mass graves   Vincent described the steadily increasing deaths in London:
'Now the Grave doth open its mouth without measure. Multitudes,
multitudes, in the valley of the shadow of death thronging daily

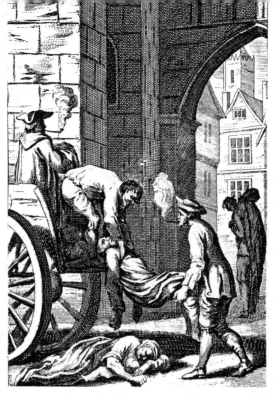

Plague victims are 'carted off' by men smoking to avoid infection

into Eternity; the Churchyards now are stuft so full with dead corpses, that they are in many places swell'd two or three foot higher than they were before, and new ground is broken up to bury the dead (53).'

When the burials became too many for the churchyards, large pits were dug, as described by Defoe: 'Into these pits they had put perhaps fifty or sixty bodies each; then they made larger holes, wherein they buried all that the cart brought in a week, which, by the middle to the end of August, came to from 200 to 400 a week; and they could not well dig them larger, because of the order of the magistrates confining them to leave no bodies within six feet of the surface; and the water coming on at about seventeen or eighteen feet, they could not well, I say, put more in one pit (54).'

Men came round at night with carts crying, 'Bring out your dead!', to take the bodies of plague victims to the pits. Defoe told of one drunken street-musician who was carted away for burial by John Hayward, under-sexton of St Stephen's, Coleman Street: 'As soon as the cart stopped the fellow awaked and struggled a

A narrow escape

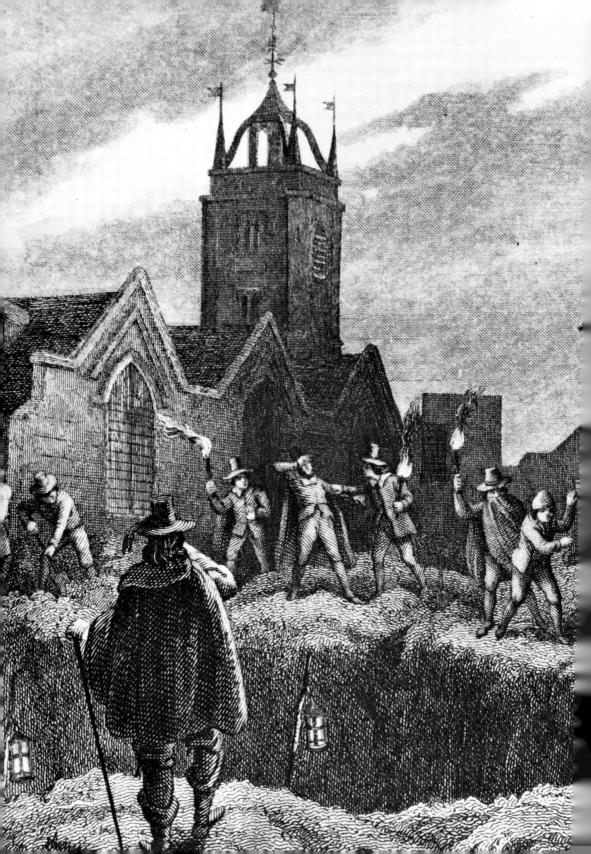

little to get his head out from among the dead bodies, when, raising himself up in the cart, he called out, "Hey! where am I?" This frighted the fellow that attended about the work; but after some pause John Hayward, recovering himself, said, "Lord bless us! There's somebody in the cart not quite dead!" So another called to him and said, "Who are you?" The fellow answered, "I am the poor piper. Where am I?" "Where are you?" says Hayward. "Why, you are in the dead-cart, and we are going to bury you." "But I an't dead though, am I?" says the piper, which made them laugh a little, though, as John said, they were heartily frighted at first; so they helped the poor fellow down, and he went about his business (55).'

When Sir Robert Long, an auditor in the Exchequer, left London in July, he wrote these instructions to his clerk about the care of his town house: 'Lett noe body stirre out, nor any suitors come into the house or office.

One man's precautions

'Lett every one take every morning a little London treacle, or the kernel of a walnutt, with five leaves of rue and a grayne of salt beaten together and roasted in a figg, and soe eaten; and never stirre out fasting.

'Lett not the porter come into the house; take all course you can agaynst the ratts, and take care of the catts; the little ones that will not stirre out may be kept, the great ones must be killed or sent away (56).'

A Cambridge undergraduate wrote to his tutor on 18 July about conditions in London: 'Blessed be the lord I got to London safe on Wensday by eleven of the clock and there is but very little notice tooke of the sickness in London though the bills are very great. There dyd threescore and 18 in St Giles in the feild scince the bill, and 5 in one hour in parish scince. It spreads very much. I went by many houses in London that were shut up—all over the city almost. Nobody that is in London feares to goe anywhere but in St Giles's. They have a bellman there with a cart. There dye so many that the bell would hardly ever leave ringing and so they ring not at all. The citizens begin to shut up apace; nothing hinders them from it but fear of the houses breaking open. My fathers has beene shut up about a weeke, but theyr is hardly an house open in the Strand, nor the Exchange. The sickness is at Tottenham high

A student's letter

Facing page The great pit in Aldgate, London, one of the mass graves dug during 1665

crosse but Mr Moyse would not have you let his son know. It is much at Hogsden, so that I saw them as I went in the road ly in a small thackt house, and I believe all most starved so great a dread it strikes into the people. I tarryd in London till Thursday in the afternoon because the tide would not serve, but then went to Windsor (57).'

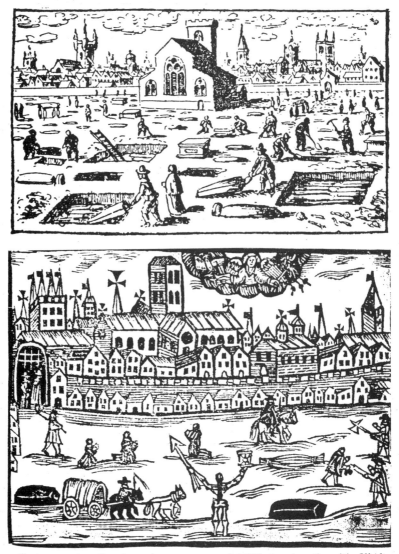

Cartoons on a London plague poster of 1665 showing the city filled with death

4 The Worst Days of All

Height of the Plague

THROUGHOUT the hot summer John Evelyn recorded in his diary the growing figures of deaths from the *Bills of Mortality* (58).

'*On 16th July:* There died of the plague in London this weeke 1,100, and in the weeke following above 2,000. Two houses were shut up in our parish.

'*On 8th August:* Died this week in London 4,000.'

'*On 15th August:* There perished this week 5,000.'

A day of fasting and penitence was appointed on 2 August; Evelyn went to church to hear his Vicar preach: 'A solemn fast thro' England to deprecate God's displeasure against the land by pestilence and war; our Dr. preaching on 26 Levit: 41, 42. that the meanes to obtaine remission of punishment was not to repine at it, but humbly submit to it (59).'

Pepys' dream

On an August evening, Pepys recalled a dream about himself and a noted beauty of the court and then came across the body of a victim of the Plague: 'Up by 4 o'clock and walked to Greenwich, where called at Captain Cocke's and to his chamber, he being in bed, where something put my last night's dream into my head, which I think is the best that ever was dreamt, which was that I had my Lady Castlemayne in my armes; and then dreamt that this could not be awake, but that it was only a dream: but that since it was a dream, and that I took so much real pleasure in it, what a happy thing it would be if when we are in our graves (as Shakespeere resembles it) we could dream, and dream but such dreams as this, that then we should not need to be so fearful of death as we are this plague time. By water to the Duke of Albemarle, with whom I spoke a great deale in private. It was dark

The Diseases and Casualties this Week.

Disease	Count	Disease	Count
Abortive	4	Imposthume	8
Aged	45	Infants	22
Bleeding	1	Kingsevil	4
Broken legge	1	Lethargy	1
Broke her scull by a fall in the street at St. Mary Woolchurch	1	Livergrown	1
		Meagrome	1
		Palsie	1
Childbed	28	Plague	4237
Chrisomes	9	Purples	2
Consumption	126	Quinsie	5
Convulsion	89	Rickets	23
Cough	1	Rising of the Lights	18
Dropsie	53	Rupture	1
Feaver	348	Scurvy	3
Flox and Small-pox	11	Shingles	1
Flux	1	Spotted Feaver	166
Frighted	2	Stilborn	4
Gowt	1	Stone	2
Grief	3	Stopping of the stomach	17
Griping in the Guts	79	Strangury	3
Head-mould-shot	1	Suddenly	2
Jaundies	7	Surfeit	74
		Teeth	111
		Thrush	6
		Tissick	9
		Ulcer	1
		Vomiting	10
		Winde	4
		Wormes	20

Christned { Males — 90, Females — 81, In all — 171 }
Buried { Males — 2777, Females — 2791, In all — 5568 } Plague — 4237

Increased in the Burials this Week — 249
Parishes clear of the Plague — 27   Parishes Infected — 103

The Assize of Bread set forth by Order of the Lord Maior and Court of Aldermen, A penny Wheaten Loaf to contain Nine Ounces and a half, and three half-penny White Loaves the like weight.

'The Diseases and Casualties this Week', showing 4,237 plague deaths out of a total of 5,568

before I could get home, and so land at Churchyard stairs, where to my great trouble I met a dead corps of the plague in the narrow ally just bringing down a little pair of stairs. But I thank God I was not much disturbed at it. However, I shall beware of being late abroad again (60).'

Dr Boghurst

William Boghurst, a doctor who worked heroically among the sick, advertised in the *Intelligencer* on 31 July his medicines which he was prepared to sell cheaply: 'Whereas William Boghurst, Apothecary at the White Hart in St Giles, in the Fields, hath

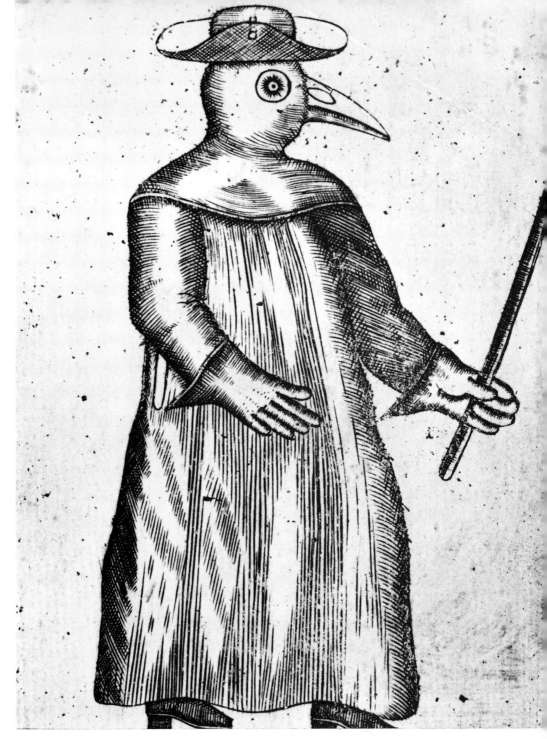

A plague doctor. His birdlike head covering, perfumed inside, is designed
to combat infection

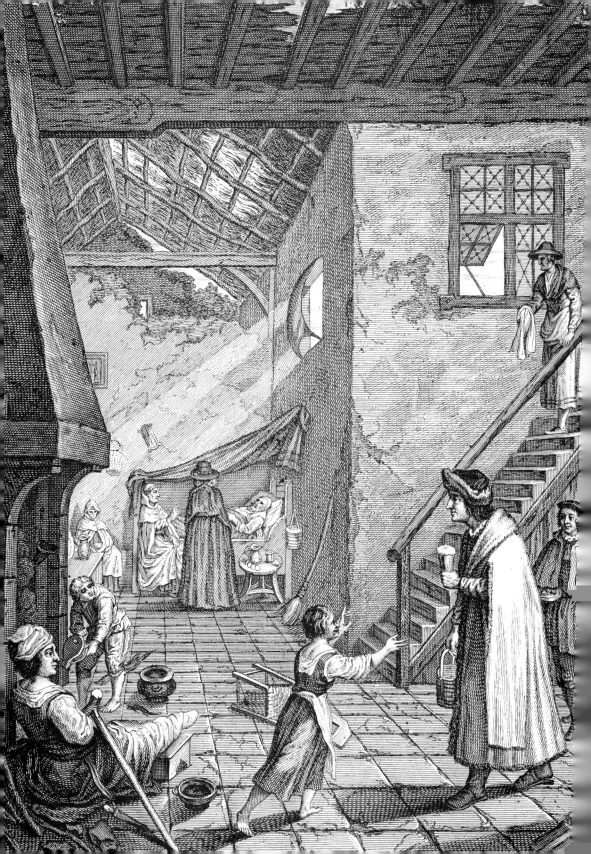

administered a long time to such as have been infected with the Plague; to the number of forty, fifty or sixty patients a day, with wonderful success, by God's blessing upon certain excellent medicines which he hath, as a Water, a Lozenge, etc.

'Also an Electuary Antidote, of but 8*d.* the ounce price. This is to notify that the said Boghurst is willing to attend any person informed and desiring his attendance, either in City, Suburbs or Country, upon reasonable terms, and that the remedies above mentioned are to be had at his house or shop, at the White Hart aforesaid (61).'

Nathaniel Hodges, another selfless doctor, described how he visited the sick in their homes: 'Entring their Houses, I immediately had burnt some proper Thing upon Coals, and also kept in my mouth some Lozenges all the while I was examining them ... I took Care not to go into Rooms of the Sick when I sweated, or were short-breathed with Walking; and kept my Mind as composed as possible, being sufficiently warned by such who had grievously suffered by Uneasiness in that Respect (62).'

Dr Hodges

After his visits, Hodges was kept busy by people who came to him for advice often until nine o'clock in the evening: 'I then concluded the Evening at Home, by drinking Chearfulness of my old favourite Liquor, which encouraged Sleep, and an easier Breathing through the Pores all Night (63).'

Modern scientists know that the Plague was spread by fleas carried by rats, but this was not known at the time. Indeed, the Lord Mayor ordered all dogs and cats in London to be killed, which meant that the rats increased. As Boghurst scornfully wrote: 'Sure, the rat killers will have a sweeping trade next year, the Arsenick and Ratbane being all spent, and the cats killed (64).'

Dogs, cats and rats

Pepys reflected sadly on the effect of the Plague on human nature: 'After dinner to Greenwich where I found 'my Lord Bruncker. We to walk in the Park, and there eat some fruit out of the King's garden, and thence walked home, my Lord Bruncker giving me a very neat cane to walk with; but it troubled me to pass by Coome farme where about twenty-one people have died of the plague, and three or four days since I saw a dead corps in a coffin lie in the Close unburied; and a watch is constantly kept there night and day to keep the people in, the plague making us

The Plague and human nature

Facing page Visiting plague victims

cruel as doggs one to another (65).'

Poor strangers, who caught the Plague in a parish, were often moved beyond the boundary to save the cost of sending them to the pest-house or burying them. Extracts from the accounts of St Alphage, London Wall (66):

> *Item.* Given to a man to carry away a sick man for feare hee should dye in the streete within this parish   .   .   .   .   1*s*. 0*d*.
> *Item.* Paid for carrying a sick man out of the parish to prevent further charge   .   .   .   .   1*s*. 0*d*.

In the worst-stricken parishes, family after family died in many streets. John Allin, a physician, wrote to a friend in the country: 'Never did so many Husbands and Wives dye together; never did so many Parents carry their Children with them to the Grave, and go together into the same House under Earth, who had lived together in the same House upon it. Now the nights are too short to bury the dead, the whole day (though at so great a length) is hardly sufficient to light the dead that fall therein, into their Beds. ... Death approacheth neerer and neerer, not many doores off, and the pitt open dayly within view of my chamber window. The Lord fitt mee and all of us for our last end! (67).'

As the Plague spread, new remedies were desperately tried. A pamphlet, *The Plague's Approved Physitian*, gave this advice for healing the swellings produced by the disease: '*If there doe a botch appeare:* Take a Pigeon and plucke the feathers off her taile, very bare, and set her taile to the sore, and shee will draw out the venom till she die; then take another and set too likewise, continuing so till all the venome be drawne out, which you shall see by the Pigeons, for they will die with the venome as long as there is any in (the tumour): also a chicken or henne is very good (68).'

No better was this remedy prescribed by the College of Physicians: 'Take a greate onion, hollow it, put into it a fig, rue cut small, and a dram of Venice treacle; put it close stopt in wet paper, and roast it in the embers; apply it hot unto the tumour; lay three or four, one after another; let one lie three hours (69).'

Dr Boghurst condemned the suffering caused to people by such useless remedies: 'To what purpose I do not know unless they delighted to torment people, for it put them to as much paine as if they had been on the wrack, worse than Death itself (70).'

Pepys wrote in his diary on the last day of August: 'Thus this month ends with great sadness upon the publick, through the greatness of the plague every where through the kingdom almost. In the City died this week 7,496, and of them 6,102 of the plague. But it is feared that the true number of the dead this week is near 10,000; partly from the poor that cannot be taken notice of through the greatness of the number, and partly from the Quakers and others that will not have any bell ring for them (71).'

Pepys liked to dress well, and even amid the Plague he had thoughts like this: 'Up; and put on my coloured silk suit very fine, and my new periwigg, bought a good while since but durst not wear because the plague was in Westminster when I bought it; and it is a wonder what will be the fashion after the plague is done as to periwiggs, for nobody will dare to buy any haire for fear of the infection, that it had been cut off of the heads of people dead of the plague (72).'

Early in September Pepys saw the great bonfires which were set alight in the streets in a vain attempt to purify the air of infection: 'Busy all the morning writing letters to several, so to dinner, to London, to pack up more things thence: and there I looked into the street and saw fires burning in the street, as it is through the whole City, by the Lord Mayor's order. Thence by water to the Duke of Albemarle's: all the way fires on each side of the Thames, and strange to see in broad daylight two or three burials upon the Banke-side, one at the very heels of another: doubtless all of the plague, and yet at least forty or fifty people going along with every one of them (73).'

Defoe worked out the cost of the fires. A 'chalder' or 'chaldron' was about 28 cwts and, owing to sickness among the seamen on the coal-ships from Tyneside, cost about £40 at the height of the Plague: 'The public fires which were made on these occasions, as I have calculated it, must necessarily have cost the city about 200 chalders of coals a week, if they had continued, which was indeed a very great quantity; but as it was thought necessary, nothing was spared. However, as some of the physicians cried them down, they were not kept alight above four or five days (74).'

As a member of the Vestry of Greenwich, Pepys agreed that

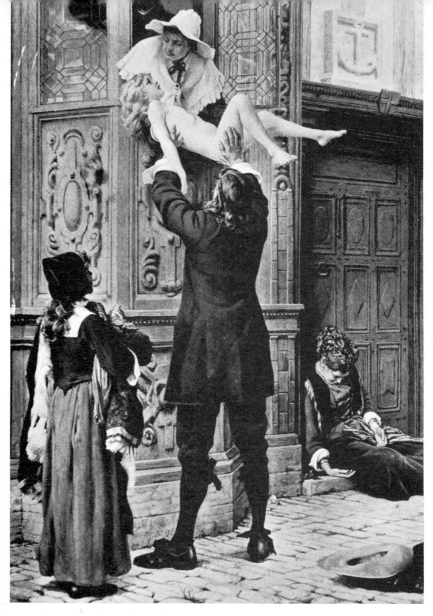

Frank Topham's famous painting, 'Rescued from the Plague'

A child saved   one particular child should be allowed to remain there, though
refugees from London were usually sent back. By 'Gracious Street'
he meant 'Gracechurch Street' in the City of London: 'Among
other stories one was very passionate, methought, of a complaint
brought against a man in the towne for taking a child from London

from an infected house. Alderman Hooker told us it was the child of a very able citizen in Gracious Street, a saddler, who had buried all the rest of his children of the plague, and himself and wife now being shut up and in despair of escaping, did desire only to save the life of this little child; and so prevailed to have it received stark-naked into the arms of a friend, who brought it (having put it into new fresh clothes) to Greenwich; where upon hearing the story, we did agree it should be permitted to be received and kept in the town (75).'

Pepys recorded also how the Vestry of Greenwich tried to stop people crowding to funerals, in order to lessen the spread of the infection: 'I up to the Vestry at the desire of the Justices of the Peace, in order to the doing something for the keeping of the plague from growing; but Lord! to consider the madness of the people of the town, who will (because they are forbid) come in crowds along with the dead corps to see them buried; but we agreed on some orders for the prevention thereof (76).' *Dangers of funerals*

The terror of those days was graphically described by Pepys in a letter he wrote on 4 September after he had retired to Woolwich: '... having stayed in the city till above 7400 died in one week, and of them above 6000 of the plague, and little noise heard day or night but tolling of bells; till I could walk Lombard Street and not meet twenty persons from the one end to the other and not fifty upon the Exchange; till whole families (ten or twelve together) have been swept away; till my very physician (Dr. Burnet) who undertook to secure me against any infection (having survived the month of his own being shut up) died himself of the Plague; till the nights (though much lengthened) are grown too short to conceal the burials of those that died the day before, people being thereby constrained to borrow daylight for that service; lastly till I could find neither drink nor meat safe, the butcheries being everywhere visited, my brewer's house shut up, and my baker with his whole family dead of the plague ... Greenwich begins apace to grow sickly (77).' *Pepys on the terror*

Later he jotted down his impressions of the Plague in a disjointed way: 'My meeting dead corpses of the Plague, carried to be buried close to me at noonday through the city in Fenchurch Street. To see a person sick of the sores, carried close by me by

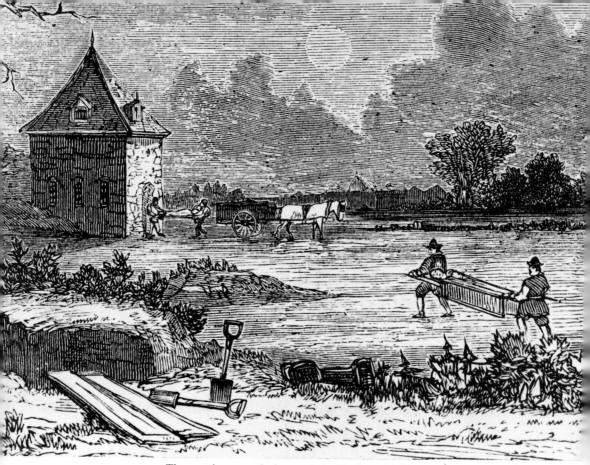

The pest-house and plague pit in Finsbury Fields, London, 1665

Gracechurch in a hackney coach. My finding the Angel Tavern at the lower end of Tower Hill shut up, and more than that the alehouse at the Tower Stairs, and more than that, that the person was then dying of the Plague when I was last there a little while ago at night. To hear that poor Payne, my waiter, had buried a child and is dying himself. To hear that a labourer I sent but the other day to Dagenhams to know how they did there, is dead of the plague, and that one of my own watermen, that carried me daily, fell sick as soon as he had landed me on Friday morning last, when I had been all night upon the water … and is now dead of the plague … And lastly that both my servants W. Hewer and Tom Edwards have lost their fathers, both in St Sepulchre parish, of the plague this week, do put me into great apprehension and melancholy and with good reason (78).'

5 The Slow Decline

IN THE MIDDLE of September Pepys feared that hopes of a decline in the Plague were false: 'Up, and after being trimmed, the first time I have been touched by a barber these twelvemonths, I think, and more, went to Sir J. Minnes's and thence to the Duke of Albemarle. But, Lord! what a sad time it is to see no boats upon the River; and grass grows all up and down White Hall court, and nobody but poor wretches in the streets! And, which is worst of all, the Duke showed us the number of the plague this week, brought in the last night from the Lord Mayor; that it is encreased about 600 more than the last, which is quite contrary to all our hopes and expectations, from the coldness of the late season (79).' *False hopes*

By October many of the poor were in a desperate condition, as Evelyn discovered: 'To London, and went thro' the whole Citty, having occasion to alight out of the coach in severall places about buisinesse of mony, when I was environ'd with multitudes of poore pestiferous creatures begging almes; the shops universaly shut up, a dreadful prospect! (80).'

By the last week of November Pepys was enquiring how many of his acquaintances were alive: 'Up, and after doing some business at the office, I to London, and there in my way, at my old oyster shop in Gracious Streete, bought two barrels of my fine woman of the shop, who is alive after all the plague, which now is the first observation or inquiry we make at London concerning everybody we knew before it (81).'

Clarendon reflected at the end of the Plague: 'The great number of those who died consisted of women and children, and the lowest and poorest sort of the people; so that, as I said before, few men missed any of their acquaintance when they returned, not many of wealth or quality or of much conversation being dead; yet some of either sort there were (82).'

'Great joy'   The end of November found Pepys at last able to feel sure that the Plague was abating: 'Great joy we have this week in the weekly Bill, it being come to 544 in all, and but 333 of the plague; so that we are encouraged to get to London soon as we can (83).'

A late death   Defoe instanced a family which died of the Plague after coming back to London that November: 'One John Cock, a barber in St Martin's-le-Grand, was an eminent example of this; I mean of the hasty return of the people when the plague was abated. This John Cock had left the town with his whole family, and locked up his house, and was gone in the country, as many others did; and finding the plague so decreased in November that there died but 905 per week of all diseases, he ventured home again. He had in his family ten persons; that is to say, himself and wife, five children, two apprentices, and a maid-servant. He had not been returned to his house above a week, and began to open his shop and carry on his trade, but the distemper broke out in his family, and within about five days they all died, except one; that is to say, himself, his wife, all his five children, and his two apprentices; and only the maid remained alive (84).'

Indeed, Sir George Downing wrote from London in December: 'People come to town and tumble over the goods and household stuff in infected houses during this sickness, which occasions the lengthening out of the malady (85).'

The king   Defoe recorded the return of the King and the more gradual
returns   return of the courtiers: 'The Court, indeed, came up soon after Christmas, but the nobility and gentry, except such as depended upon and had employment under the administration, did not come so soon (86).'

The diarists   This was the last entry by Evelyn in his diary for the year 1665:
give thanks   'Now blessed be God for his extraordinary mercies and preservation of me this yeare, when thousands and ten thousands perish'd and were swept away on each side of me, there dying in our parish this yeare 406 of the pestilence! (87).'

Pepys wrote in his diary on the same day: 'Thus ends this year, to my great joy, in this manner. I have raised my estate from

£1,300 in this year to £4,000. I have got myself great interest, I think, by my diligence, and my employments increased by that of Treasurer of Tangier and Surveyor of the Victuals. It is true we have gone through great melancholy because of the Great Plague, and I put to great charges by it, by keeping my family long at Woolwich, and myself and another part of my family, my clerks, at my charge at Greenwich, and a maid at London (88).'

On 5 January 1666, Pepys noted that people were beginning to return to London again: 'I with my Lord Bruncker and Mrs Williams by coach with four horses to London to my Lord's house in Covent-Guarden. But Lord! what staring to see a nobleman's coach come to town. And porters every where bow to us, and such begging of beggars! And a delightfull thing it is to see the towne full of people again as now it is; and shops begin to open, though in many places seven or eight together and more all shut, but yet the towne is full compared with what it used to be: I mean the City end, for Covent-Guarden and Westminster are yet very empty of people, no Court nor gentry being there (89).'

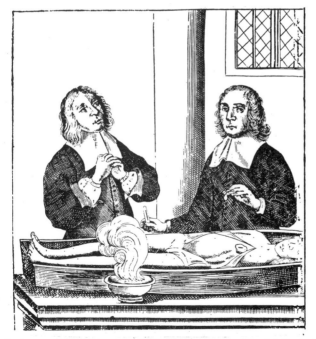

Frontispiece to *The Mannere of Bissecting the Pestillential Body* (1666) showing surgeons carrying out an autopsy on a plague victim

Defoe gave an account of the reception given to doctors and clergymen, who returned to London after having fled the Plague: 'Great was the reproach thrown on those physicians who left their patients during sickness, and now they came to town again nobody cared to employ them. They were called deserters, and frequently bills were set up upon their doors and written, "Here is a doctor to be let," so that several of those physicians were fain for a while to sit still and look about them, or at least remove their dwellings, and set up in new places and among new acquaintance. The like was the case with the clergy, whom the people were indeed very abusive to, writing verses and scandalous reflections upon them, setting upon the church-door, "Here is a pulpit to be let," or sometimes, "to be sold," which was worse (90).'

On Sunday 4 February 1666, Pepys, for the first time since the Plague, went to church, where he heard a poor excuse and a bad sermon: 'My wife and I the first time together at church since the Plague, and now only because of Mr Mills his coming home to preach his first sermon; expecting a great excuse for his leaving the parish before anybody went, and now staying till all are come home; but he made but a very poor and short excuse, and a bad sermon. It was a frost, and had snowed last night, which covered the graves in the churchyard, so as I was the less afraid for going through (91).'

Baxter estimated the number who died from the Plague in London: 'The number that died in London (besides all the rest of the land) was about an hundred thousand, reckoning the Quakers and others, that were never put in the bills of mortality, with those that were in the bills (92).'

Dr Gumble, who saw all the official reports sent to Albemarle, thought that as many again died when the Plague spread to the rest of England: 'This Judgment the next year took its circuit, and visited many great Cities and Towns in the Nation, so that in 1665 and 1666 there died about two hundred thousand persons of men, women and children of the pestilence, which was a visitation beyond any formerly in this Nation; and I hope and pray that God will never send the like, and that we nor our Posterity after us may never feel such another Judgment (93).'

People continued to fear another outbreak of plague for the rest of the seventeenth century. An item of account from a fashionable lady's housekeeping-book in 1698: 'June 19. Ingredients had by Mistress Monroe for Plague Water, 1*s*. 1*d*. (94).'

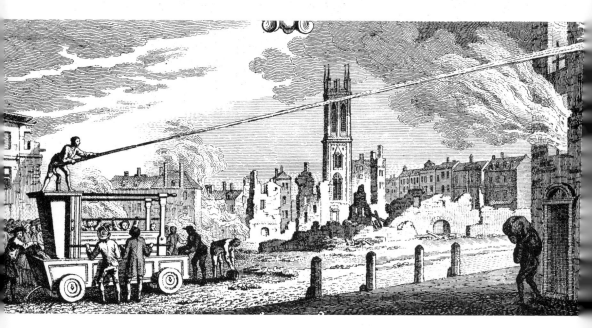

A fire engine

6 The Outbreak of the Fire

FIRES were not uncommon in seventeenth-century London. In 1633, for instance, part of London Bridge was destroyed. Nehremiah Wallington, a turner living in the City, wrote about it: 'Yet the timber, and the wood, and the coals in the cellars, could not be quenched all that week, till the Tuesday following, in the afternoon, the 19 February, for I was there myself, and had a live coal of fire in my hand, and burnt my finger with it. Notwithstanding there were as many night and day as could labour one by another, to carry away timber, and bricks, and tiles, and rubbish cast down into the lighters. So that on Wednesday the Bridge was cleared that passengers might go over (95).'

The fire of 1633

Yet as late as 1657, James Howell wrote confidently of London's fire defences. The new fire-engines were hand squirts which proved useless: 'There's no place ... better armed against the fury of the fire; for besides the pitched Buckets that hang in the Churches and Halls, there are divers new Engines for that pupose (96).'

Clarendon told how the Fire began early on the morning of Sunday, 2 September 1666: 'It was upon the first day of that September, in the dismal year of 1666, (in which many prodigies were expected, and so many really fell out,) that that memorable and terrible fire brake out in London, which begun about midnight, or nearer the morning of Sunday, in a baker's house at the end of Thames-street next the Tower, there being many little narrow alleys and very poor houses about the place where it first appeared; and then finding such store of combustible materials, as that street is always furnished with in timber-houses, the fire prevailed so powerfully, that that whole street and the neighbourhood was

How the fire began

59

Overleaf A model of London Bridge as it appeared before the Great Fire

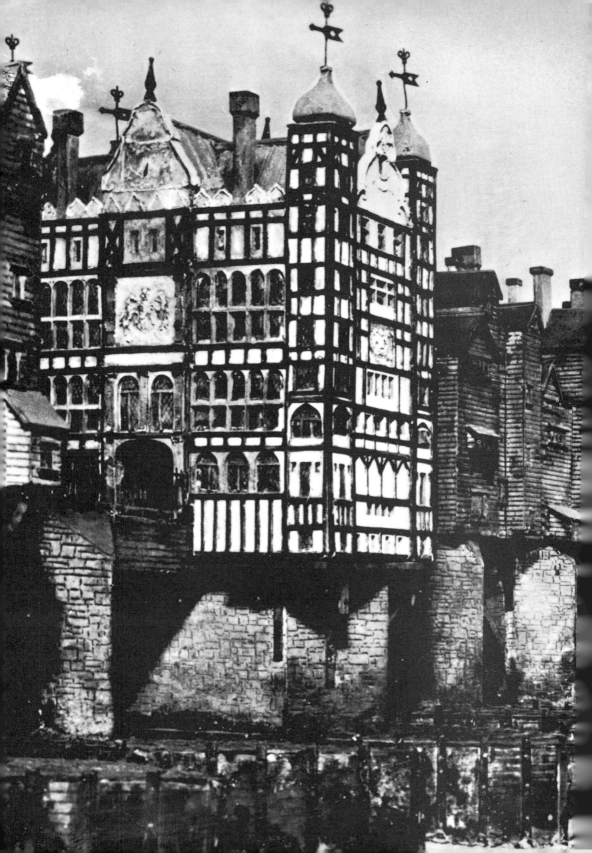

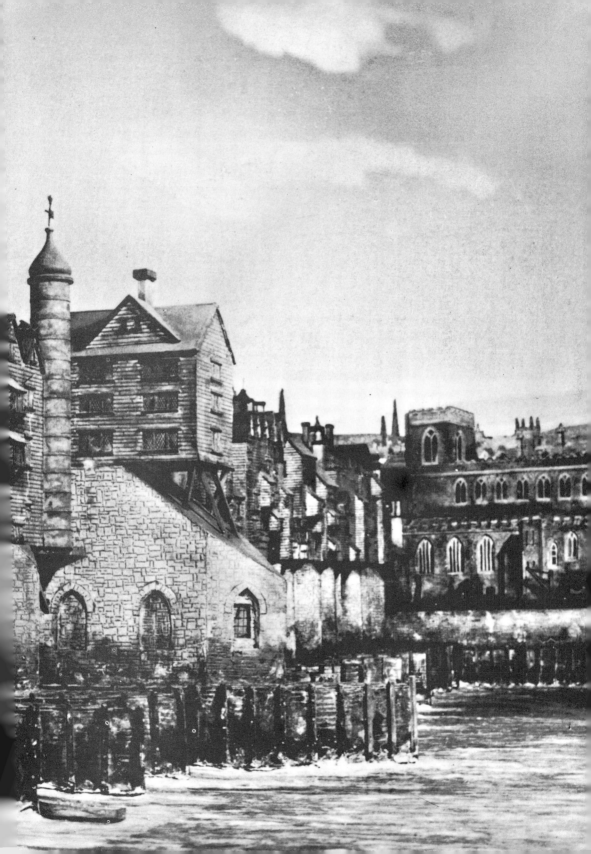

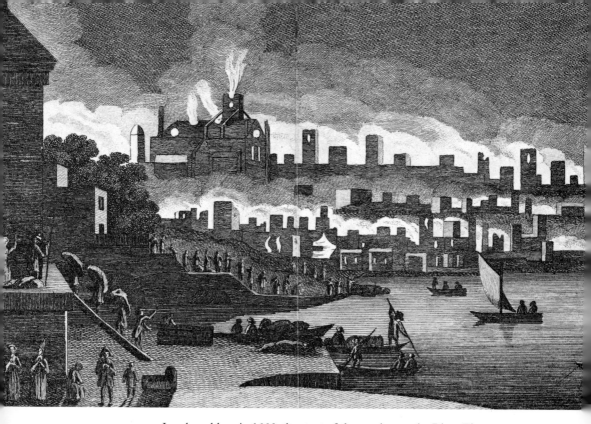

London ablaze in 1666, the start of the exodus on the River Thames

in so short a time turned to ashes, that few persons had time to save and preserve any of their goods; but were a heap of people almost as dead with the sudden distraction, as the ruins were which they sustained (97).'

William Burnet (afterwards Bishop of Salisbury), then a preacher in London, remembered that the Fire broke out before the City had recovered from the Plague: 'To complete the miseries of this year, no sooner was the plague so abated in London that the inhabitants began to return to their houses, than a most dreadful fire, on the 2nd of September, broke out in the City, and raged for three days, as if it had commission to devour everything that was in its way. Above twelve thousand houses were burnt down, with the greatest part of the furniture and merchandise that were in them (98).'

Pepys was told early on Sunday morning about the Fire by a

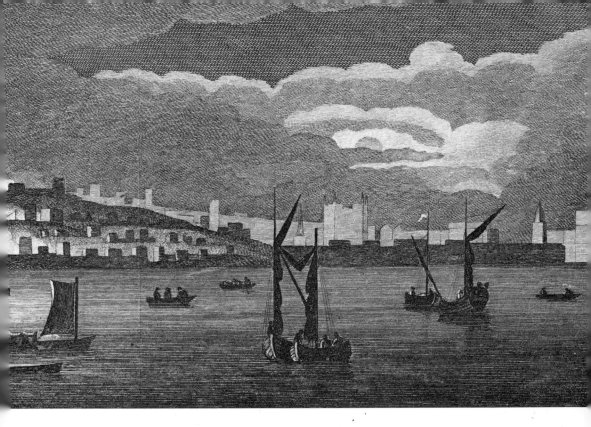

maidservant, but it did not cause him any alarm: 'Some of our
mayds sitting up late last night to get things ready against our
feast to-day, Jane called us up about three in the morning to tell
us of a great fire they saw in the City. So I rose and slipped on my
night-gowne and went to her window, and thought it to be on the
back-side of Marke-lane at the farthest; but, being unused to such
fires as followed, I thought it far enough off; and so went to bed
again to sleep (99).'

When he got up, the Fire, though farther from his house, was
spreading: 'About seven rose again to dress myself, and there
looked out of the window and saw the fire not so much as it was,
and farther off. So to my closett to set things to rights after yesterday's cleaning. By and by Jane comes and tells me that she hears
that above 300 houses have been burned down to-night by the fire
we saw, and that it is now burning down all Fish-street, by London
Bridge (100).'

Overleaf Refugee boats crowding the firelit Thames

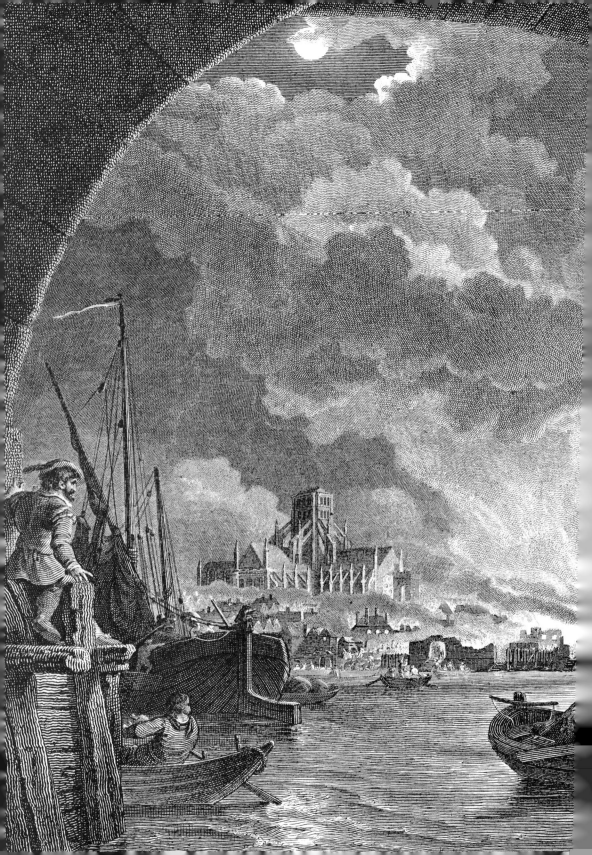

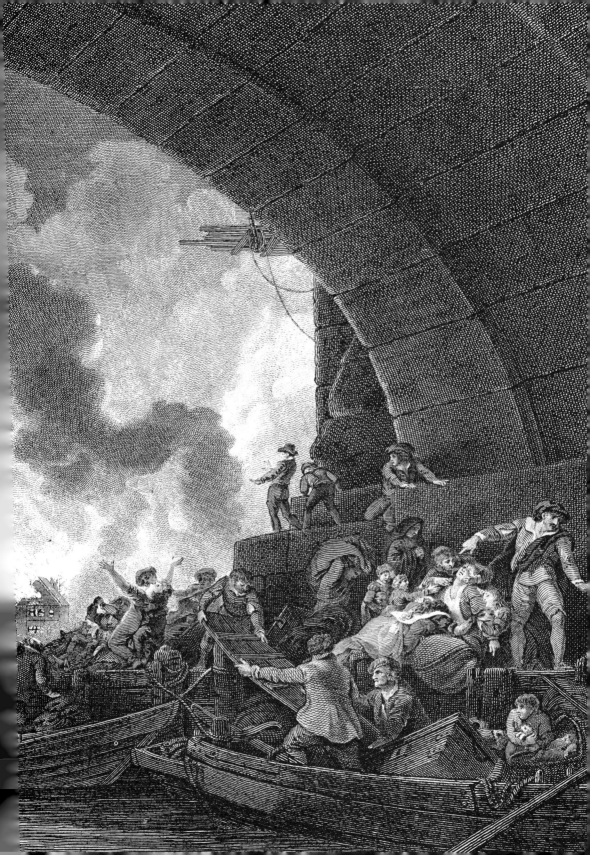

He went out and discovered the full extent and horror of the Fire: 'So I made myself ready presently and walked to the Tower, and there got up upon one of the high places, Sir J. Robinson's little son going up with me; and there I did see the houses at that end of the bridge all on fire, and an infinite great fire on this and the other side the end of the bridge. So with my heart full of trouble, I down to the water-side, and there got a boat and through bridge, and there saw a lamentable fire. Poor Michell's house, as far as the Old Swan, already burned that way, and the fire running further. Everybody endeavouring to remove their goods, and flinging into the river or bringing them into lighters that lay off; poor people staying in their houses as long as till the very fire touched them, and then running into boats, or clambering from one pair of stairs by the water-side to another. And among other things the poor pigeons, I perceive, were loth to leave their houses, but hovered about the windows and balconys till they were, some of them burned, their wings, and fell down (101).'

A fifteen-year-old schoolboy, William Taswell, first heard about the Fire when attending Morning Prayer at Westminster Abbey: 'On Sunday, between ten and eleven forenoon, as I was standing upon the steps which lead up to the pulpit in Westminster Abbey, I perceived some people below me running to and fro in a seeming disquietude and consternation; immediately almost a report reached my ears that London was in conflagration; without any ceremony I took leave of the preacher, and having ascended Parliament Steps, near the Thames, I soon perceived four boats crowded with objects of distress. They had escaped from the fire scarce under any covering except that of a blanket (102).'

On Pepys' advice, it was decided to pull down houses in the hope of halting the Fire: 'Having staid, and in an hour's time seen the fire rage every way, and nobody, to my sight, endeavouring to quench it, but to remove their goods and leave all to the fire; and having seen it get as far as the Steele-yard, and the wind mighty high and driving it into the City, and every thing after so long a drought proving combustible, even the very stones of churches, I to White Hall and there up to the King's closett in the Chappell, where people come about me and I did give them an account dismayed them all, and word was carried in to the King. So I was called for and did tell the King and Duke of Yorke what I saw, and that unless his Majesty did command houses to be pulled down nothing could stop the fire. They seemed much troubled, and the King commanded me to go to my Lord Mayor from him and command him to spare no houses, but to pull down before the fire every way. The Duke of York bid me tell him that if he would have any more soldiers he shall (103).'

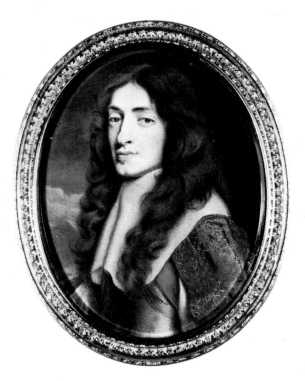

James, Duke of York

Pepys observed that everyone's first aim was to save their possessions: 'Here meeting with Captain Cocke, I in his coach which he lent me, and Creed with me to Paul's, and there walked along Watling-street as well as I could, every creature coming away loaden with goods to save, and here and there sicke people carried away in beds. Extraordinary good goods carried in carts and on backs (104).'

Goods and chattels

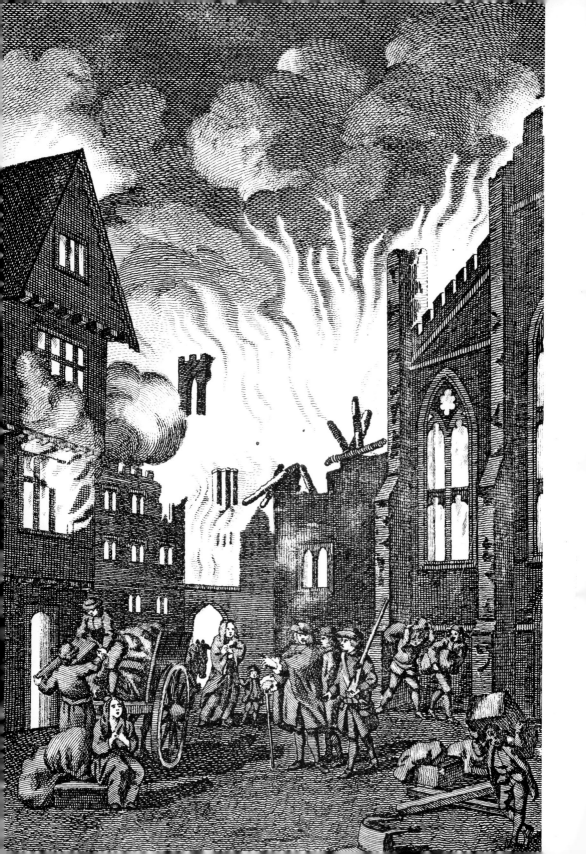

He found the Lord Mayor overwhelmed by the situation: 'At last met my Lord Mayor in Canning-street like a man spent, with a handkercher about his neck. To the King's message he cried, like a fainting woman, "Lord! what can I do? I am spent: people will not obey me. I have been pulling down houses, but the fire overtakes us faster than we can do it." That he needed no more soldiers; and that, for himself, he must go and refresh himself, having been up all night. So he left me, and I him, and walked home, seeing people all almost distracted; and no manner of means used to quench the fire. The houses, too, so very thick thereabouts, and full of matter for burning, as pitch and tarr, in Thames-street; and warehouses of oyle, and wines, and brandy and other things. I saw Mr. Isaake Houblon, the handsome man, prettily dressed and dirty, at his door at Dowgate receiving some of his brothers' things, whose houses were on fire; and, as he says have been removed twice already, and he doubts (as it soon proved) that they must be in a little time removed from his house also, which was a sad consideration. And to see the churches all filling with goods by people who themselves should have quietly been there at this time (105).'

In the afternoon, Pepys found the Fire spreading and the con- fusion growing: 'By this time it was about twelve o'clock; and so home, and soon as dined, away and walked through the City, the streets full of nothing but people and horses and carts loaden with goods. They now removing out of Canning-streete (which received goods in the morning) into Lumbard-streete, and further. Met with the King and Duke of York in their barge, and with them to Queen-hithe, and there called Sir Richard Browne to them. Their order was only to pull down houses apace; and so below bridge at the water-side, but little was or could be done, the fire coming upon them so fast. River full of lighters and boats taking in goods, and good goods swimming in the water, and only I observed that hardly one lighter or boat in three that had the goods of a house in, but there was a pair of Virginalls in it (106).'

The *London Gazette* gave the official account of the failure to stop the flames by demolishing houses: 'Many attempts were made to prevent the spreading of it by pulling down houses, and making great intervals, but all in vain, the fire seising upon the

Facing page Last minute efforts to save possessions

timber and rubbish and so continuing itself, even through those spaces and raging in a bright flame all Monday and Tuesday (107).'

Foreign sabotage ? Clarendon described how popular suspicion found foreign scapegoats for the Fire. He should have said 'Sunday' instead of 'Monday': 'Monday morning produced first a jealousy, and then as universal conclusion, that this fire came not by chance nor did they care where it began; but the breaking out in several places at so great distance from each other made it evident, that it was by conspiracy and combination. And this determination could not hold long without discovery of the wicked authors, who were concluded to be all the Dutch and all the French in the town, though they had inhabited the same places above twenty years. All of that kind, or, if they were strangers, of what nation so-ever, were laid hold of; and after all the ill usage that can consist in words, and some blows and kicks, they were thrown into prison (108).'

Roman Catholic sabotage ? Then, according to Clarendon, suspicion included the Roman Catholics: 'And shortly after, the same conclusion comprehended all the Roman Catholics, the papists, who were in the same predicament of guilt and danger, and quickly found that their only safety consisted in keeping within doors; and yet some of them, and of quality, were taken by force out of their houses, and carried to prison (109).'

Dr Denton, the King's Physician, was certain the Roman Catholics were responsible and wrote in a letter: 'It is generally beleeved, but not at court, that the Papists have designed this & more, many & strong presumptions there are for it, as gunpowder, & balls & wildfire taken about many of them, that if they destroy them there are more left behind to doe the business; send them to Whitehall they are all dismissed (110).'

The mob Taswell's account of the effect of the fear and suspicion: 'A blacksmith in my presence, meeting an innocent Frenchman walking along the street, felled him instantly to the ground with an iron bar. I could not help seeing the innocent blood of this exotic flow in a plentiful stream down to his ankles. In another place I saw the incensed populace divesting a French painter of all the goods he had in his shop; and, after having helped him off with many other things, levelling his house to the ground under this pretence, namely, that they thought himself was desirous of setting his own house on fire, that the conflagration might become more general (111).'

As the afternoon passed, Pepys found the Fire spreading faster than ever: 'Having seen as much as I could now, I away to White Hall by appointment, and there walked to St. James's Parke, and there met my wife and Creed, and walked to my boat; and there upon the water again, and to the fire up and down, it still encreasing, and the wind great. So near the fire as we could for smoke; and all over the Thames, with one's face in the wind, you were almost burned with a shower of fire-drops. This is very true; so as houses were burned by these drops and flakes of fire, three or four, nay, five or six houses, one from another (112).'

As darkness fell, he watched the terrible sight from the River: 'When we could endure no more upon the water, we to a little ale-house on the Bankside, over against the Three Cranes, and there staid till it was dark almost, and saw the fire grow; and, as it grew darker, appeared more and more, and in corners and upon steeples, and between churches and houses as far as we could see up the hill of the City, in a most horrid malicious bloody flame, not like the fine flame of an ordinary fire. We staid till, it being darkish, we saw the fire as only one entire arch of fire from this to the other side the bridge, and in a bow up the hill for an arch of above a mile long: it made me weep to see it. The churches, houses and all on fire and flaming at once; and a horrid noise the flames made, and the cracking of houses at their ruine (113).'

Before that terrible Sunday was over, Pepys found his own house menaced by the creeping flames: 'So home with a sad heart, and there find poor Tom Hater come with some few of his goods saved out of his house, which is burned. I invited him to lie at my house and did receive his goods, but was deceived in his lying there, the newes coming every moment of the growth of the fire; so as we were forced to begin to pack up our owne goods and prepare for their removal; and did by moonshine (it being brave dry and moonshine and warm weather) carry much of my goods into the garden, and Mr Hater and I did remove my money and iron chests into my cellar, as thinking that the safest place. And got my bags of gold into my office ready to carry away, and my chief papers of accounts also there, and my tallys into a box by themselves. So

Pepys watches the fire

Pepys' house in danger

71

great was our fear, as Sir W. Batten hath carts come out of the country to fetch away his goods this night. We did put Mr Hater, poor man, to bed a little; but he got but very little rest, so much noise being in my house taking down of goods (114).'

7 · The Fire at its Height

ON MONDAY MORNING, Evelyn viewed the Fire with foreboding from Southwark: 'I had public prayers at home. The fire continuing, after dinner I took coach with my wife and sonn and went to the Bank side in Southwark, where we beheld the dismal spectacle, the whole Citty in dreadfull flames neare the water side; all the houses from the Bridge, all Thames Street, and upwards towards Cheapeside, downe to the Three Cranes, were now consum'd: and so returned exceedinge astonished what would become of the rest (116).'

Evelyn

Clarendon recorded how the Fire continued unabated until the wind dropped, which was really on Tuesday afternoon and not Wednesday as he wrongly remembered: 'The fire and the wind continued in the same excess all Monday, Tuesday, and Wednesday, till afternoon, and flung and scattered brands burning into all quarters; the nights more terrible than the days, and the light the same, the light of the fire supplying that of the sun (115).'

Clarendon

Meanwhile, Pepys had been up early to move his possessions: 'About four o'clock in the morning my Lady Batten sent me a cart to carry away all my money and plate and best things to Sir W. Rider's at Bednall-greene: which I did, riding myself in my night-gowne in the cart, and, Lord! to see how the streets and the highways are crowded with people running and riding, and getting of carts at any rate to fetch away things. I find Sir W. Rider tired with being called up all night and receiving things from several friends. His house full of goods, and much of Sir W. Batten's and Sir W. Pen's. I am eased at my heart to have my treasure so well secured (117).'

Pepys moves house

73

Overleaf The Fire of London, painted by Lieven Verschuur

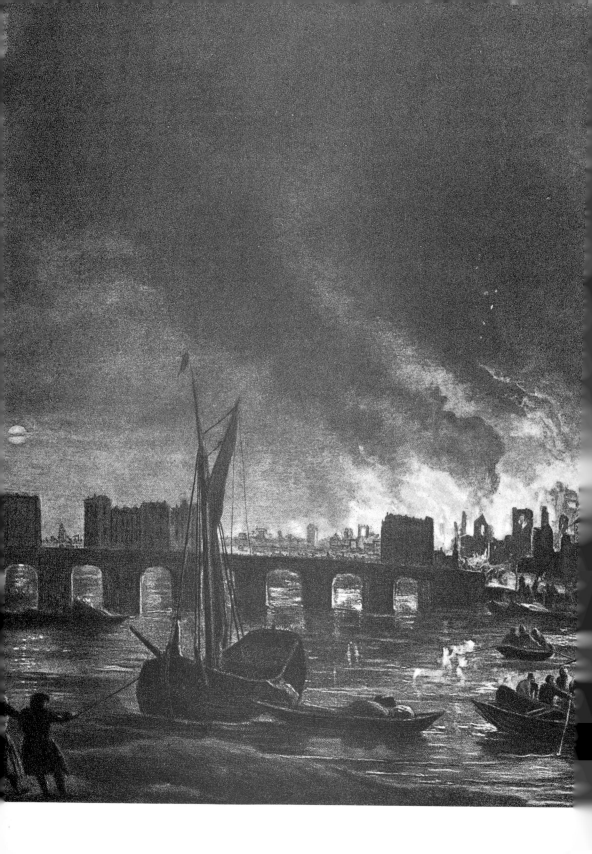

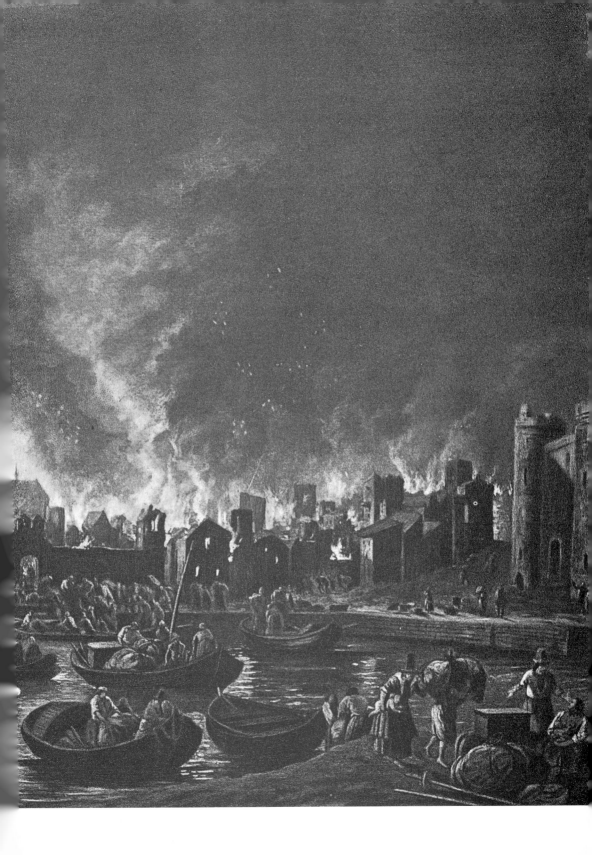

As an important naval official, he was in close contact with the Duke of York, the Lord High Admiral, who now directed the fire-fighting operations: 'Then home, with much ado to find a way, nor any sleep all this night to me nor my poor wife, but then, and all this day, she and I and all my people labouring to get away the rest of our things. The Duke of Yorke come this day by the office and spoke to us, and did ride with his guard up and down the City to keep all quiet (he being now Generall, and having the care of all) (118).'

Lady Hobart
Lady Hobart wrote from Chancery Lane to Sir Ralph Verney on Monday morning: 'Poor London is almost burnt out. It began on Saturday night and has burnt ever since, and is at this time more fierce than ever, it did begin in Pudding Lane at a bakers, where a Dutch rogue lay ... 'Tis thought Fleet Street will be burnt by tomorrow, there is nothing left in any house there, nor in the Temple ... 'Tis the Dutch who fire, there was one taken in Westminster setting his outhouse on fire and they have attempted to fire many places and there is an abundance taken with grenades and powder! ... I am almost out of my wits, we have packed up all our goods and cannot get a cart for money, they give five and ten pound for carts, I cannot get one for twenty pound to go out of town ... and I fear I shall lose all I have and must run away (119).'

Pepys'
servants run
away
Even during the Fire, Pepys and his wife had on Monday evening one of their numerous troublesome incidents with their maidservants: 'This day, Mercer being not at home but against her mistress's order gone to her mother's, and my wife going thither to speak with W. Hewer met her there, and was angry; and her mother saying that she was not a 'prentice girl, to ask leave every time she goes abroad, my wife with good reason was angry, and when she came home bid her be gone again. And so she went away, which troubled me; but yet less than it would, because of the condition we are in fear of coming into in a little time of being less able to keepe one in her quality. At night lay down a little upon a quilt of W. Hewer's in the office, all my owne things being packed up or gone; and after me my poor wife did the like, we having fed upon the remains of yesterday's dinner, having no fire nor dishes, nor any opportunity of dressing any thing (120).'

76   *Panic*
Clarendon observed the panic that the uncertainty aroused in

many people: 'And indeed whoever was an eyewitness of that terrible prospect, can never have so lively an image of the last conflagration till he beholds it; the faces of all people in a wonderful dejection and discomposure, not knowing where they could repose themselves for one hour's sleep, and no distance thought secure from the fire, which suddenly started up before it was suspected; so that people left their houses and carried away their goods from many places which received no hurt, and whither they afterwards returned again; all the fields full of women and children, who had made a shift to bring thither some goods and conveniences to rest upon, as safer than any houses, where yet they felt such intolerable heat and drought, as if they had been in the middle of the fire (121).'

Evelyn saw how helpless everyone seemed to be: 'The conflagration was so universal, and the people so astonish'd, that from the beginning, I know not by what despondency or fate, they hardly stirr'd to quench it, so that there was nothing heard or seene but crying out and lamentation, running about like distracted creatures, without at all attempting to save even their goods; such a strange consternation there was upon them, so as it burned both in breadth and length, the Churches, Public Halls, Exchange, Hospitals, Monuments, and ornaments, leaping after a prodigious manner from house to house and streete to streete, at greate distances one from the other; for the heate with a long set of faire and warme weather had even ignited the aire and prepar'd the materials to conceive the fire, which devour'd after an incredible manner houses, furniture, and every thing (122).'

Richard Baxter afterwards wrote in much the same way: 'The season had been exceeding dry before, and the wind in the east, where the fire began. The people having none to conduct them aright could do nothing to resist it, but stand and see their houses burn without remedy, the engines being presently out of order and useless. The streets were crowded with people and carts, to carry away what goods they could get out. And they that were most active and befriended (by their wealth) got carts, and saved much; and the rest lost almost all. The loss in houses and goods is scarcely to be valued (123).'

Clarendon said that the country people were more sympathetic *Country people* towards Londoners during the Fire than they had been in the Plague: 'The country sent in carts to help those miserable people who had saved any goods: and by this means, and the help of coaches, all the neighbour villages were filled with more people than they could contain, and more goods than they could find room for; so that those fields became likewise as full as the other about London and Westminster (124).'

Brick and wood

He also recorded that the newer, brick houses resisted the Fire better than the older, wooden ones: 'It was observed that where the fire prevailed most, when it met with brick buildings, if it was not repulsed, it was so well resisted that it made a much slower progress; and when it had done its worst, that the timber and all the combustible matter fell, it fell down to the bottom within the house, and the walls stood and enclosed the fire, and it was burned out without making a further progress in many of those places; and then the vacancy so interrupted the fury of it, that many times the two or three next houses stood without much damage (125).'

Whole streets ablaze

Vincent wrote: 'If you opened your eye to the opening of the streets, where the Fire was come, you might see in some places whole streets at once in flames, that issued forth as if they had been so many great Forges from the opposite windows, which folding together, were united into one great flame throughout the whole street; and then you might see the Houses tumble, tumble, tumble, from one end of the street to the other with a great crash, leaving the foundations open to the view of the heavens (126).'

Evelyn watched the City burning on Monday night: 'The fire having continu'd all this night (if I may call that night which was light as day for ten miles round about, after a dreadfull manner) when conspiring with a fierce Eastern wind in a very drie season; I went on foote to the same place, and saw the whole South part of the City burning from Cheapeside to the Thames, and all along Cornehill (for it likewise kindl'd back against the wind as well as forward), Tower Streete, Fen-church Streete, Gracious Streete, and so along to Bainard's Castle, and was now taking hold of St. Paule's Church, to which the scaffolds contributed exceedingly (127).'

Vincent saw how, on Monday night, four great lines of flame converged at the eastern end of Cheapside: 'All these four joyning together, break into one great flame at the corner of Cheapside with such a dazzling light, and burning heat, and roaring noise by the fall of so many houses together that was very amazing (128).'

An Italian wrote after the Fire: 'One would need to have been a Nero to have watched such a spectacle without pity ... Men, women and children of all ages and of all ranks, ran through the streets, their backs loaded with their most precious goods; and among them were carried many sick and disabled persons, who had been driven from their houses by the fire ... As they ran they made a heartrending murmur ... the miseries of this people were appalling (129).'

Evelyn found the River Thames full of refugees: 'Here we saw the Thames cover'd with goods floating, all the barges and boates laden with what some had time and courage to save, as, on the

Refugees

Contemporary print of London during the height of the Fire

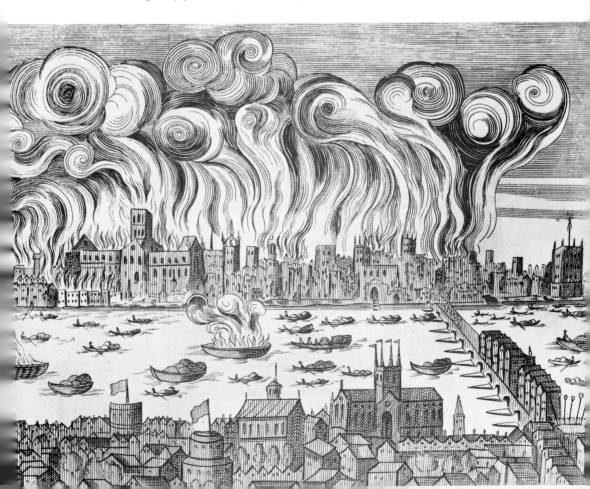

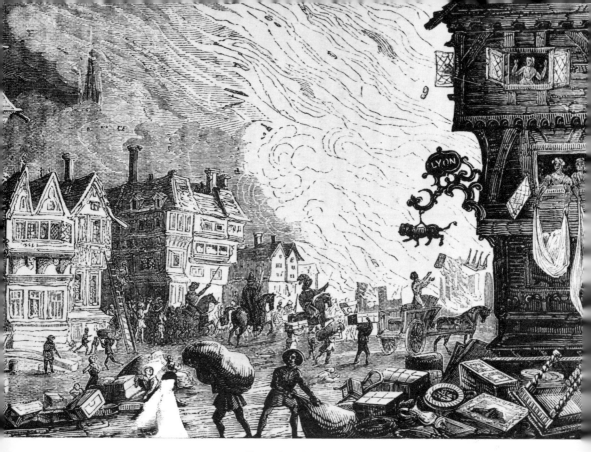

Chaos in London's burning streets

other, the carts, &c. carrying out to the fields, which for many miles were strew'd with moveables of all sorts, and tents erecting to shelter both people and what goods they could get away (130).'

An inferno　　He wrote of the scene that evening: 'Oh the miserable and calamitous spectacle! such as happly the world had not seene the like since the foundation of it, nor be outdon till the universal conflagration of it. All the skie was of a fiery aspect, like the top of a burning oven, and the light seene above 40 miles round about for many nights. God grant mine eyes may never behold the like, who now saw above 10,000 houses all in one flame; the noise and cracking and thunder of the impetuous flames, the shrieking of women and children, the hurry of people, the fall of Towers, Houses and Churches, was like an hideous storme, and the aire all about so hot and inflam'd that at the last one was not able to approach it, so that they were forc'd to stand still and let the flames burn on, which they did for neere two miles in length and one in bredth. The clowds also of smoke were dismall and reach'd upon computation neer 56 miles in length (131).'

So he went home, fearing that London would be no more: 'Thus I left it this afternoone burning, a resemblance of Sodom, or the last day. It forcibly call'd to my mind that passage—*non enim hic habemus stabilem civitatem*: the ruines resembling the picture of Troy. London was, but is no more! Thus I returned home (132).'

On Tuesday morning Pepys saw to the safety of the rest of his possessions: 'Up by break of day to get away the remainder of my things. Sir W. Batten not knowing how to remove his wine did dig a pit in the garden and laid it in there; and I took the opportunity of laying all the papers of my office that I could not otherwise dispose of. And in the evening Sir W. Pen and I did dig another and put our wine in it, and I my Parmazan cheese as well as my wine and some other things (133).' *Pepys' ingenious idea*

Vincent described the destruction of Cheapside, London's widest thoroughfare, at daybreak on Tuesday: 'Cheapside is alight in a few hours time; many fires meeting there, as in the centre; from Sopar Lane, Bow Lane, Bread Street, Friday Street and Old Cheape, the fire comes up almost together and breaks furiously into Broad Street, and most of that side of the way was together in flames, a dreadful spectacle! And then partly by the fall of houses across the way, the other side is so quickly kindled, and doth not stand long after (134).' *Cheapside*

Evelyn described the Fire on Tuesday, when the Fire was at its height: 'The burning still rages, and it was now gotten as far as the Inner Temple; all Fleet Streete, the Old Bailey, Ludgate Hill, Warwick Lane, Newgate, Paules Chaine, Watling Streete, now flaming, and most of it reduc'd to ashes; the stones of Paules flew like granados, the mealting lead running downe the streetes in a streame, and the very pavements glowing with fiery rednesse, so as no horse nor man was able to tread on them, and the demolition had stopp'd all the passages, so that no help could be applied. The Eastern wind still more impetuously driving the flames forward. Nothing but the Almighty power of God was able to stop them, for vaine was the help of man (135).' *Terrible Tuesday*

Overleaf A detailed model of the Great Fire of London

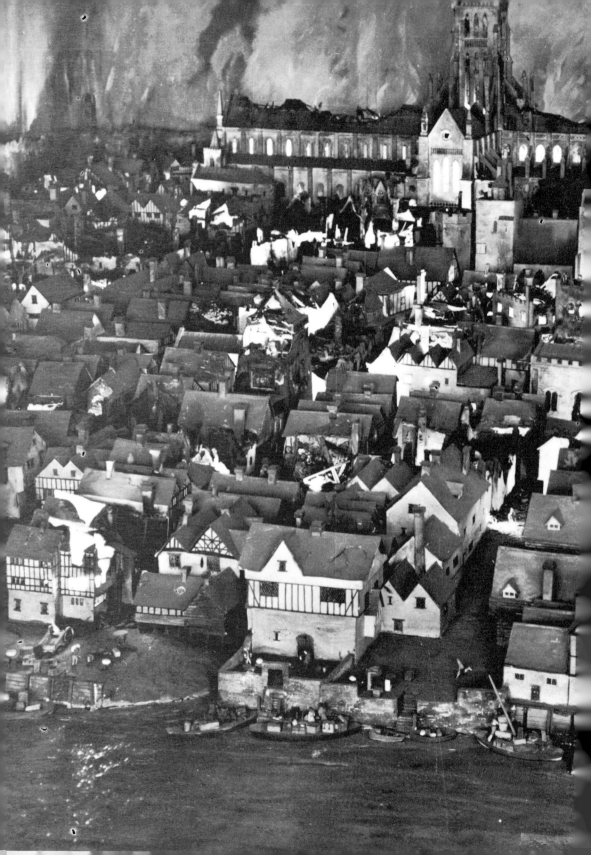

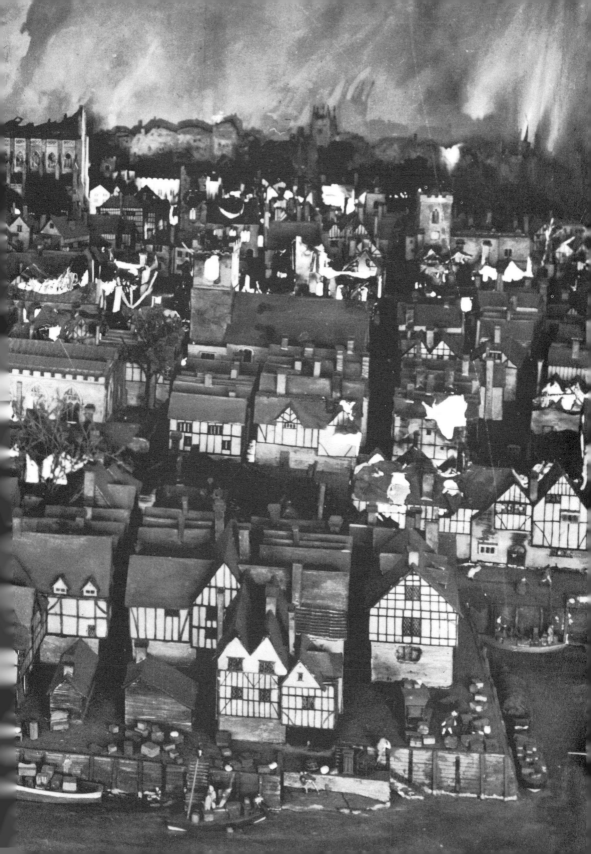

Gunpowder
versus fire He thought that the blowing up of houses by gunpowder would have been done earlier but for opposition from influential City men: 'It crossed towards Whitehall; but oh, the confusion there was then at that Court! It pleas'd his Majesty to command me among the rest to looke after the quenching of Fetter Lane end, to preserve if possible that part of Holborn whilst the rest of the gentlemen tooke their several posts, some at one part, some at another (for now they began to bestir themselves, and not till now, who hitherto had stood as men intoxicated, with their hands acrosse) and began to consider that nothing was likely to put a stop but the blowing up of so many houses as might make a wider gap than any had yet ben made by the ordinary method of pulling them downe with engines; this some stout seamen propos'd early enough to have sav'd nearly the whole Citty, but this some tenacious and avaritious men, aldermen, &c. would not permitt, because their houses must have ben of the first (136).'

Pepys gets
help On Tuesday afternoon, Pepys sought the help of workmen from the naval dockyards to save his office: 'This afternoon, sitting melancholy with Sir W. Pen in our garden, and thinking of the certain burning of this office without extraordinary means, I did propose for the sending up of all our workmen from Woolwich and Deptford yards (none whereof yet appeared), and to write to Sir W. Coventry to have the Duke of Yorke's permission to pull down houses rather than lose this office, which would much hinder the King's business. So Sir W. Pen he went down this night, in order to the sending them up to-morrow morning; and I wrote to Sir W. Coventry about the business, but received no answer (137).'

A hospital in
danger As Commissioner for Sick Seamen, Evelyn was especially anxious to save St. Bartholomew's Hospital: 'It was therefore now commanded to be practic'd, and my concerne being particularly for the Hospital of St. Bartholomew neere Smithfield, where I had my wounded and sick men, made me the more diligent to promote it; nor was my care for the Savoy lesse (138).'

The fiery sky Despite a cheerful supper, Pepys was growingly alarmed by the intensity of the Fire: 'This night Mrs. Turner (who, poor woman, was removing her goods all this day, good goods into the garden, and knows not how to dispose of them) and her husband supped with my wife and I at night in the office, upon a shoulder of mutton from the cook's, without any napkin or any thing, in a sad manner, but were merry. Only now and then walking into the garden, and saw how horridly the sky looks, all on a fire in the night, was enough to put us out of our wits; and indeed it was extremely dreadful, for it looks just as if it was at us, and the whole heaven on fire. I after supper walked in the darke down to Tower-streete, and there saw it all on fire (139).'

Evelyn was relieved when the wind fell: 'It now pleas'd God by abating the wind, and by the industrie of the people, when almost all was lost, infusing a new spirit into them, that the furie of it began sensibly to abate about noone, so as it came no farther than the Temple Westward, nor than the entrance of Smithfield North: but continu'd all this day and night so impetuous toward Cripplegate and the Tower as made us all despaire; it also brake out againe in the Temple, but the courage of the multitude persisting, and many houses being blown up, such gaps and desolations were soone made, as with the former three days consumption, the back fire did not so vehemently urge upon the rest as formerly. There was yet no standing neere the burning and glowing ruines by neere a furlongs space (140).' *The wind drops*

The end of the day for Pepys—people were frightened by the blowing up of houses near the Tower because they thought its guns *Houses blown up*

St Bartholomew's Hospital in Evelyn's day

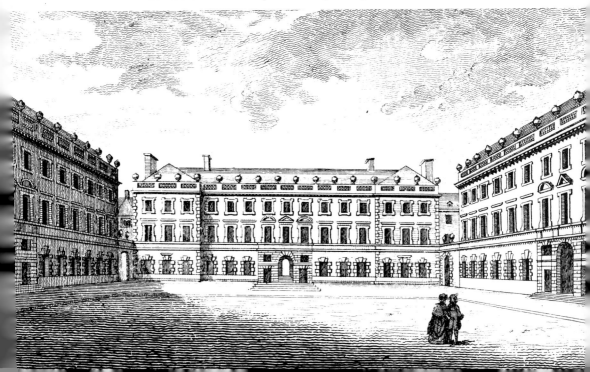

were being fired at their houses to demolish them quickly: 'Now begins the practice of blowing up of houses in Tower-streete, those next the Tower, which at first did frighten people more than any thing. W. Hewer this day went to see how his mother did, and comes late home, telling us how he hath been forced to remove her to Islington, her house in Pye-corner being burned: so that the fire is got so far that way, and all the Old Bayly, and was running down to Fleete-Streete; and Paul's is burned, and all Cheapside. I wrote to my father this night, but the post-house being burned, the letter could not go (141).'

Evelyn explained why it was vital to stop the flames reaching the Tower of London. 'Graff' means a 'ditch' or 'moat': 'In the mean time his Majesty got to the Tower by water, to demolish the houses about the graff, which being built intirely about it, had they taken fire and attack'd the White Tower where the magazine of powder lay, would undoubtedly not only have beaten downe and destroyed all the bridge, but sunke and torne the vessels in the river, and render'd the demolition beyond all expression for several miles about the countrey (142).'

Westminster Abbey and Whitehall in danger

The King feared the Fire would spread down the Strand to Whitehall and Westminster Abbey. Clarendon again should have said 'Tuesday' instead of 'Wednesday': 'On Wednesday morning, when the king saw that neither the fire decreased nor the wind lessened, he even despaired of preserving Whitehall, but was more afraid of Westminster-abbey. But having observed by his having visited all places, that where there were any vacant places between the houses, by which the progress of the fire was interrupted, it changed its course and went to the other side; he gave order for pulling down many houses about Whitehall, some whereof were newly built and hardly finished, and sent many of his choice goods by water to Hampton-Court; as most of the persons of quality in the Strand, who had the benefit of the river, got barges and other vessels, and sent their furniture for their houses to some houses some miles out of town. And very many on both sides the Strand, who knew not whither to go, and scarce what they did, fled with their families out of their houses into the streets, that they might not be within when the fire fell upon their houses (143).'

Clarendon told how the Fire stopped before burning the wealthy houses in the Strand: 'But it pleased God, contrary to all expecta- tion, that on Wednesday [really Tuesday], about four or five of the clock in the afternoon, the wind fell: and as in an instant the fire decreased, having burned all on the Thames side to the new build- ings of the Inner Temple next to Whitefriars, and having consumed them, was stopped by that vacancy from proceeding further into that house; but laid hold on some old buildings which joined to Ram-alley, and swept all those into Fleet-street. And the other side being likewise destroyed to Fetter-lane, it advanced no further; but left the other part of Fleet-street to the Temple-bar, and all the Strand, unhurt, but what damage the owners of the houses had done to themselves by endeavouring to remove; and it ceased in all other parts of the town near the same time: so that the greatest care then was, to keep good guards to watch the fire that was upon the ground, that it might not break out again (144).'

He recalled how Charles now gave orders for food supplies to be brought into London: 'When the night, though far from being a quiet one, had somewhat lessened the consternation, the first care the king took was, that the country might speedily supply markets in all places, that they who had saved themselves from burning might not be in danger of starving; and if there had not been extraordinary care and diligence used, many would have perished that way. The vast destruction of corn, and all other sorts of provisions, in those parts where the fire had prevailed, had not only left all that people destitute of all that was to be eat or drank; but the bakers and brewers, which inhabited the other parts which were unhurt, had forsaken their houses, and carried away all that was portable: insomuch as many days passed, before they were enough in their wits and in their houses to fall to their occupations; and those parts of the town which God had spared and preserved were many hours without anything to eat, as well as they who were in the fields. And yet it can hardly be conceived, how great a supply of all kinds was brought from all places within four and twenty hours (145).'

A firefighter afterwards wrote of the scene on Tuesday night, when the wind rose again for a short time: 'Night coming on, the flames increased by the wind rising, which appeared to us so ter- rible to see, from the very ditch the shore quite up to the Temple

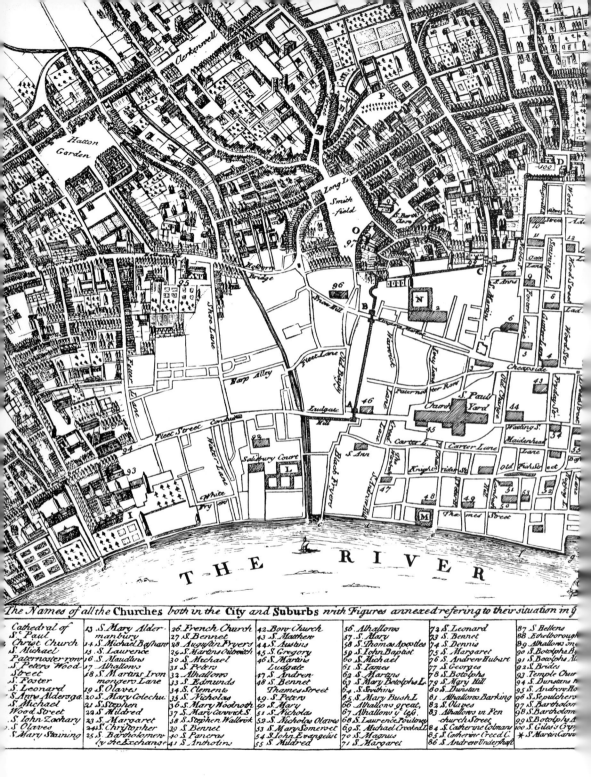

The Names of all the **Churches** both in the **City** and **Suburbs** with Figures annexed refering to their situation in ye

Cathedral of S.ᵗ Paul	13 S. Mary Alder-manbury	26 French Church	42 Bow-church
Christ Church	14 S. Michael Basham	27 S. Bennet	43 S. Matthew
S. Michael Paternoster-row	15 S. Laurence	28 Augustin Fryers	44 S. Austins
S. Peters Wood-Street	16 S. Maudlins	29 S. Martins Oitwich	45 S. Gregory
S. Foster	17 Alhallows	30 S. Michael	46 S. Martins Ludgate
S. Leonard	18 S. Martins Iron-mongers Lane	31 S. Peters	47 S. Andrew
S. Anns Aldersga.	19 S. Olaves	32 Alhallows	48 S. Bennet Thames Street
S. Michael Wood Street	20 S. Mary Colechu.	33 S. Edmunds	49 S. Peters
S. John Zachary	21 S. Stephen	34 S. Clements	50 S. Mary
S. Olaves	22 S. Mildred	35 S. Nicholas	51 S. Nicholas
S. Mary Staining	23 S. Margaret	36 S. Mary Woodnoth	52 S. Nicholas Olaves
	24 S. Chrystopher	37 S. Mary Canwick S.	53 S. Mary Somerset
	25 S. Bartholomew by the Exchange	38 S. Stephen Walbrock	54 S. John Evangelist
		39 S. Bennet	55 S. Mildred
		40 S. Pancras	
		41 S. Antholins	

56 Alhallows	74 S. Leonard	87 S. Hellens
57 S. Mary	73 S. Bennet	88 S. Ethelborough
58 S. Thomas Apostles	74 S. Dennis	89 Alhallows in
59 S. John Baptist	75 S. Margaret	90 S. Botolphs B
60 S. Michael	76 S. Andrew Hubart	91 S. Bocolphs Al
61 S. James	77 S. Georges	92 S. Brides
62 S. Martins	78 S. Botolphs	93 Temple Chur
63 S. Mary Botolphs L.	79 S. Mary Hill	94 S. Dunstans in
64 S. Swithins	80 S. Dunstan	95 S. Andrew Ho
65 S. Mary Bush L.	81 Alhallows Barking	96 S. Sepulchers
66 Alhallows great,	82 S. Olaves	97 S. Bartholom
67 Alhallows ye leß.	83 Alhallows in Pen	98 S. Bartholom
68 S. Laurence Poultney	84 S. Catherine Colmans	99 S. Botolphs A
69 S. Michael Crooked L.	85 S. Catherine Creed C.	100 S. Giles Cryp
70 S. Magnus	86 S. Andrew Undershaft	✴ S. Martin Canw
71 S. Margaret		

A contemporary plan of London immediately after the Fire, showing
virtually no buildings left standing in the heart of the City

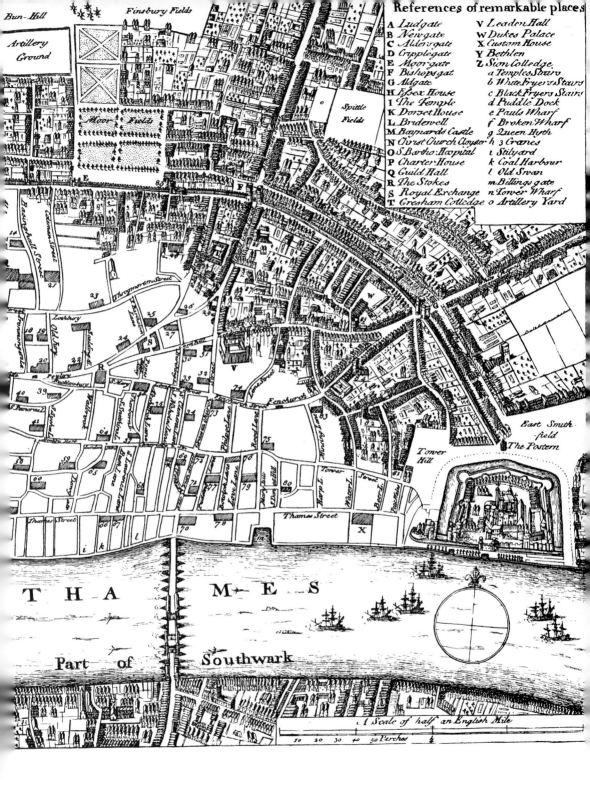

A Ludgate   V Leaden Hall
B Newgate   W Dukes Palace
C Aldersgate   X Custom House
D Cripplegate   Y Bethlen
E Moorgate   Z Sion Colledge
F Bishopsgat   a Temples Stairs
G Aldgate   b White Fryers Stairs
H Essex House   c Black Fryers Stairs
I The Temple   d Puddle Dock
K Dorset House   e Pauls Wharf
L Bridewell   f Broken Wharf
M Baynards Castle   g Queen Hyth
N Christ Church Cloyster   h 3 Cranes
O S. Bartho Hospital   i Stilyard
P Charter House   k Coal Harbour
Q Guild Hall   l Old Swan
R The Stokes   m Billings gate
S Royal Exchange   n Tower Wharf
T Gresham Colledge   o Artillery Yard

Bun-Hill   Finsbury Fields

Artillery Ground

Moor Fields

Spittle Fields

East Smith field
The Postern

Tower Hill

THAMES

Part of Southwark

A Scale of half an English Mile
10   20   30   40   50 Perches

all in a flame, and a very great breadth. At ten o'clock at night we left Somerset House, where they began to pull down some houses in hopes to save Whitehall ... Nothing can be like unto the distraction we were in, but the Day of Judgment (146).'

The end of St Paul's
Vincent tells of the destruction of St Paul's Cathedral: 'The church, though all of stone outward, though naked of houses about it, and though so high above all buildings in the City, yet within a while doth yield to the violent assaults of the conquering flames, and strangely takes Fire at the top; now the Lead melts and runs down, as if it had been snow before the Sun; and the great-beams and massy stones, with a great noise, fall upon the Pavement, and break through into Faith Church underneath; now great flakes of stone scale, and peel off strangely from the side of the Walls (147).'

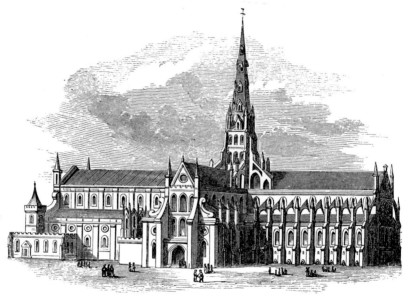

Taswell also saw St Paul's burn: 'Just after sunset at Night I went to the royal bridge (landing stage) in New Palace Yard at Westminster to take a fuller view of the fire. The people who lived contiguous to St Paul's church raised their expectations greatly concerning the absolute security of that place upon account of the immense thickness of its walls and its situation; built in a large

Above Old St Paul's Cathedral
Facing page St Paul's Cathedral in flames

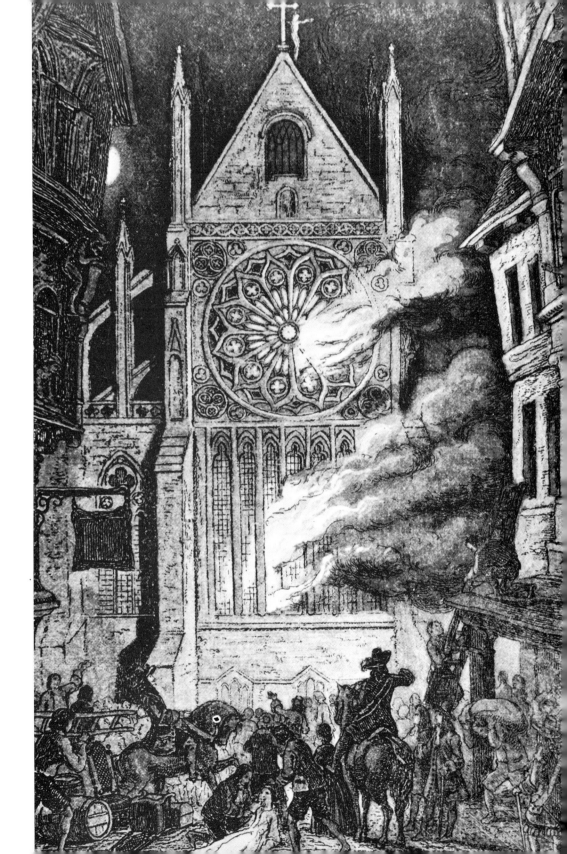

piece of ground, on every side remote from houses. Upon this account they filled it with all sorts of goods, and besides, in the church of St Faith's, under that of St Paul's, they deposited libraries of books because it was entirely arched all over; and with great caution and prudence every the least avenue through which the smallest spark might penitrate was stopped up. But this precaution availed them little. As I stood upon the bridge among others, I could not but observe the gradual approach of the fire towards that venerable fabric. About eight o'clock it broke out on the top of St Paul's Church, already scorched by the violent heat of the air, and lightning too, and before nine blazed so conspicious as to enable me to read very clearly a sixteen mo edition of Terence which I carried in my pocket (148).'

Guildhall destroyed   Vincent described the burning of the Guildhall on the Tuesday evening: 'All through the night Guild Hall was a fearful spectacle, which stood the whole body of it together in view, for several hours together, after the fire had taken it, without the flames (I suppose because the timber was such solid Oake) in a bright shining coal, as if it had been a Palace of Gold, or a Great Building of burnished Brass (149).'

8 The Quenching and the Aftermath

EARLY ON WEDNESDAY morning, his wife told Pepys that the Fire *The fire* had reached Allhallows Barking Church, nearly opposite the end *chases Pepys* of Seething Lane where they lived: 'I lay down in the office again upon W. Hewer's quilt, being mighty weary and sore in my feet with going till I was hardly able to stand. About two in the morning my wife calls me up and tells me of new cryes of fire, it being come to Barkeing Church, which is the bottom of our lane (150).'

So he decided to take his wife and gold to safety: ' I up, and finding it so resolved presently to take her away, and did, and took my gold, which was about £2,350, W. Hewer and Jane down by Proundy's boat to Woolwich; but, Lord! what a sad sight it was by moone-light to see the whole City almost on fire, that you might see it plain at Woolwich as if you were by it. There when I come I find the gates shut, but no guard kept at all, which troubled me because of discourse now begun that there is plot in it and that the French had done it. I got the gates open, and to Mr Sheldon's, where I locked up my gold and charged my wife and W. Hewer never to leave the room without one of them in it, night or day. So back again, by the way seeing my goods well in the lighters at Deptford and watched well by people (151).'

On his return, he found his house had not, after all, been destroyed: 'Home, and whereas I expected to have seen our house on fire, it being now about seven o'clock, it was not. But to the fyre, and there find greater hopes than I expected; for my confidence of finding our Office on fire was such that I durst not ask any body how it was with us till I come, and saw it not burned. But going to the fire I find, by the blowing up of houses and the

93

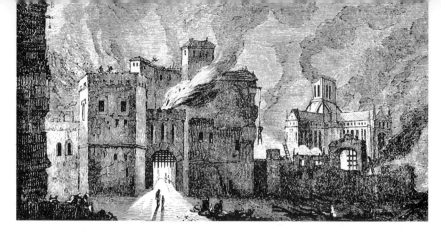

The burning of Newgate Prison, 1666

great helpe given by the workmen out of the King's yards sent up by Sir W. Pen, there is a good stop given to it, as well as at Marke-lane end as ours; it having only burned the dyall of Barking Church and part of the porch, and was there quenched (152).'

He now had time to see the havoc wrought by the Fire. By Sir Thomas Gresham's picture, he meant statue: 'I up to the top of Barking Steeple and there saw the saddest sight of desolation that I ever saw; every where great fires, oyle-cellars and brimstone and other things burning. I became afeard to stay there long, and therefore down again as fast as I could, the fire being spread as far as I could see it; and to Sir W. Pen's, and there eat a piece of cold meat, having eaten nothing since Sunday, but the remains of Sunday's dinner. And having removed all my things and received good hopes that the fire at our end is stopped, I walked into the town, and find Fanchurch-streete, Gracious-streete, and Lumbard-streete all in dust. The Exchange a sad sight, nothing standing there of all the statues or pillars but Sir Thomas Gresham's picture in the corner (153).'

He continued his walk among the scenes of destruction: 'Walked into Moorefields (our feet ready to burn, walking through the towne among the hot coles), and find that full of people, and poor wretches carrying their goods there, and every body keeping his goods together by themselves (and a great blessing it is to them that it is fair weather for them to keep abroad night and day). Drank there, and paid twopence for a plain penny loaf; thence homeward, having passed through Cheapside and Newgate Market, all burned, and seen Anthony Joyce's house in fire (154).'

On his way back home, he noticed a strange incident: 'I also did see a poor cat taken out of a hole in the chimney joyning to the wall of the Exchange, with the hair all burned off the body and yet alive. So home at night, and find there good hopes of saving our office, but great endeavours of watching all night, and having men ready; and so we lodged them in the office and had drink and bread and cheese for them. And I lay down and slept a good night about midnight (155).'

A lucky cat

Evelyn too, that Wednesday afternoon, was distressed by the plight of those whose homes had been destroyed: 'The poore inhabitants were dispers'd about St George's Fields, and Moore-fields, as far as Highgate, and severall miles in circle, some under tents, some under miserable hutts and hovells, many without a rag or any necessary utensills, bed or board, who from delicate-nesse, riches, and easy accomodations in stately and well furnish'd houses, were now reduced to extreamest misery and poverty (156).'

The homeless

The official *London Gazette* praised Charles II for his part in fighting the Fire: 'A greater instance of the affections of this City (for Charles) could never have been given than hath now been given in this sad and deplorable accident, when, if at any time, disorder might have been expected from the losses, distraction and almost desperation of some persons in their private fortunes, thousands of people not having had habitations to cover them.

Thanks to the royal family

'And yet in all this time it hath been so far from any appearance of designs or attempts against His Majesties Government, that His Majesty and his Royal Brother, out of their care to stop and prevent the fire, frequently exposing their persons with very small attendants, in all parts of the town, sometimes even to be inter-mixed with those who laboured in the business, yet nevertheless there hath not been observed so much as a murmuring word to fall from any ... beholding those frequent instances of His Majesties care of his people, forgot their own misery, and filled the streets with their prayers for His Majesty, whose trouble they seemed to compassionate before their own (157).'

Henry Griffith in a letter to his kinsman, Lord Conway, com-mended both the royal brothers, who: 'rode up and down, giving orders for blowing up of houses with gunpowder, to make void

95

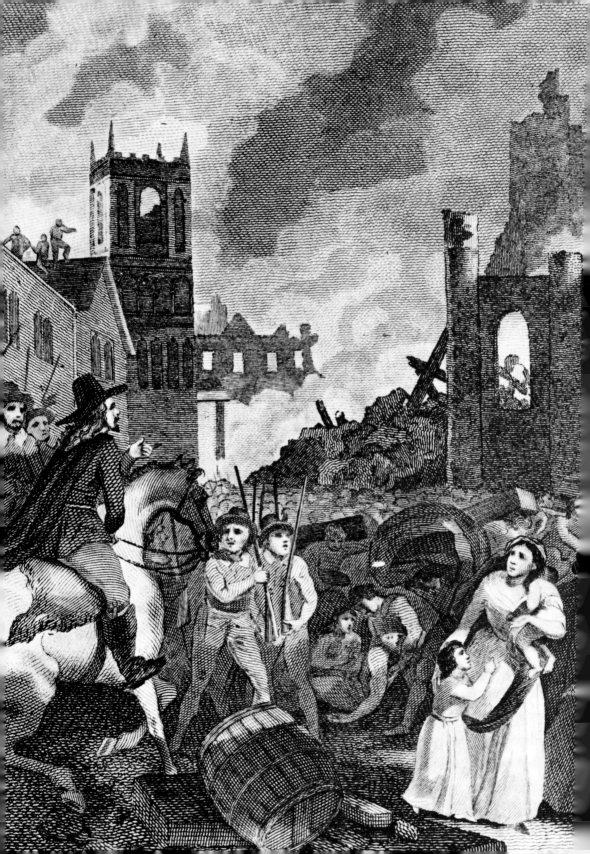

spaces for the fire to die in, and standing still to see those orders executed, exposing their persons not only to the multitude, but to the very flames themselves, and the ruins of the buildings ready to fall upon them, and sometimes labouring with their own hands to give examples to others: for which the people now do pay them, as they ought to do, all possible reverence and admiration (158).'

A quarrel

This letter describes what happened late on Wednesday night, when the Duke of York ordered the blowing up of the Paper Office to save the Middle Temple Hall: 'One of the Templars seeing gunpowder brought, came to the Duke and told him it was against the rules and charter of the Temple that any should blow that house with gunpowder, upon which Mr Germaine, the Duke's Master of the Horse, took a cudgel and beat the young lawyer to the purpose. There is no hopes of knowing who this lawyer is, but the hope that he will bring an action of battery against Mr Germaine (159).'

The hot ground

Early on Thursday morning, Taswell set out to view the ruins of St Paul's: 'On Thursday, soon after sunrising, I endeavoured to reach St Paul's. The ground so hot as almost to scorch my shoes, and the air so intensely warm that unless I had stopped some time upon Fleet Bridge to rest myself, I must have fainted under the extreme languor of my spirits. After giving myself a little time to breathe, I made the best of my way to St Paul's (160).'

Souvenirs

He found the Cathedral still burning: 'And now let any person judge of the violent emotion I was in when I perceived the metal belonging to the bells melting, the ruinous condition of its walls; whole heaps of stone of a large circumference tumbling down with a great noise just upon my feet, ready to crush me to death. I prepared myself for returning back again, having first loaded my pockets with several pieces of bell metal (161).'

Taswell sees a skeleton

And saw a gruesome sight: 'I forgot to mention that near the east walls of St Paul's a human body presented itself to me, parched up as it were with the flames, whole as to skin, meagre as to flesh, yellow as to colour. This was an old woman who fled here for safety, imagining the flames would not reach her there, Her clothes were burnt, and every limb reduced to coal (162).'

Firemen in danger

On the way back with further souvenirs, he saw several fire-engines set alight by the heat: 'In my way back I saw several

Facing page The Duke of York in charge of the fire-fighting

engines which were bringing up to its assistance all on fire, and those concerned with them escaping with great eagerness from the flames, which spread instantaneous almost like wild fire; and at last, accoutred with my sword and helmet, which I picked up among many others in the ruins, I transversed this torrid zone back again (163).'

Drinking and plundering

That same Thursday morning, Pepys set out to see the first aftermath of the Fire: 'Up about five o'clock, and there met Mr Gawden at the gate of the office to call our men to Bishop's-gate, where no fire had yet been near, and there is now one broke out. I went with the men, and we did put it out in a little time; so that that was well again. It was pretty to see how hard the women did work in the cannells, sweeping of water; but then they would scold for drink, and be as drunk as devils. I saw good butts of sugar broken open in the street, and people go and take handsfull out and put into beer and drink it (164).'

Pepys relaxes

Now he had time for clothes and food: 'And now all being pretty well I took boat and over to Southwarke, and took boat on the other side the bridge and so to Westminster thinking to shift myself, being all in dirt from top to bottom; but could not there find any place to buy a shirt or pair of gloves, Westminster Hall being full of people's goods, those in Westminster having removed all their goods; but to the Swan, and there was trimmed, and then to White Hall, but saw nobody, and so home. A sad sight to see how the River looks, no houses nor church near it, to the Temple, where it stopped. To Sir R. Ford's and there dined on an earthen platter; a fried breast of mutton; a great many of us, but very merry, and indeed as good a meal, though as ugly a one, as I ever had in my life (165).'

So Thursday ended with his fears at an end: 'Thence down to Deptford, and there with great satisfaction landed all my goods at Sir G. Carteret's safe, and nothing missed I could see, or hurt. This being done to my great content, I home and to Sir W. Batten's, and there supped well and mighty merry, and our fears over. From them to the office, and there slept with the office full of labourers, who talked and slept and walked all night long there. But strange it was to see Cloath-workers' Hall on fire these three days and nights in one body of flame, it being the cellar of oyle (166).'

A final comment by Taswell. Many booksellers had stored their books for safety in St Paul's when the Fire began: 'The papers half burnt, were carried with the wind to Eton. The Oxonians observed the rings of the sun tinged with an unusual kind of redness. A black darkness seemed to cover the whole hemisphere; and the bewailings of the people were great (167).'

Pepys mentioned the losses of the booksellers, who were perhaps the hardest hit of all the City traders: 'There is above £150,000 of books burned; all the great booksellers almost undone; not only these, but their warehouses at their Hall and under Christ-Church, and elsewhere, being all burned. A great want therefore will be of books, specially Latin books and foreign books, and, among others, the Polyglots and the new Bible, which he believes will be presently worth £40 apiece (168).'

On Friday Evelyn went to inspect the scene of the Fire: 'I went this morning on foote from White-hall as far as London Bridge, thro' the late Fleete Street, Ludgate Hill, by St. Paules, Cheapeside, Exchange, Bishopsgate, Aldersgate, and out to Moorefields, thence thro' Cornehill, &c. with extraordinary difficulty, clambering over heaps of yet smoking rubbish, and frequently mistaking where I was. The ground under my feete so hot, that it even burnt the soles of my shoes (169).'

He was especially grieved by the destruction of St Paul's Cathedral: 'At my returne I was infinitely concern'd to find that goodly Church St Paules now a sad ruine, and that beautifull portico (for structure comparable to any in Europe, as not long before repair'd by the late King) now rent in pieces, flakes of vast stone split asunder, and nothing remaining intire but the inscription in the architrave, shewing by whom it was built, which had not one letter of it defac'd. It was astonishing to see what immense stones the heate had in a manner calcin'd, so that all the ornaments, columnes, freezes, capitals and projectures of massie Portland stone flew off, even to the very roofe, where a sheet of lead covering a great space (no less than 6 akers by measure) was totally mealted; the ruines of the vaulted roofe falling broke into St Faith's, which being fill'd with the magazines of bookes belonging to the Stationers, and carried thither for safety, they were all consum'd, burning for a weeke following. It is also observable that the lead over the altar at the East end was untouch'd, and among the divers monuments, the body of one Bishop remain'd intire. Thus lay in ashes that most venerable Church, one of the most antient pieces of early piety in the Christian world, besides neere 100 more (170).'

The way the flames had consumed everthing amazed him: 'The lead, yron worke, bells, plate, &c. mealted; the exquisitely wrought Mercers Chapell, the sumptuous Exchange, the august fabriq of Christ Church, all the rest of the Companies Halls, splendid buildings, arches, enteries, all in dust; the fountaines dried up and ruin'd, whilst the very waters remain'd boiling; the voragos of subterranean cellars, wells, and dungeons, formerely warehouses, still burning in stench and dark clowds of smoke, so that in five or six miles traversing about, I did not see one loade of timber unconsum'd, nor many stones but what were calcin'd white as snow (171).'

He was also astonished by the intensity of the heat: 'The people who now walk'd about the ruines appear'd like men in some dismal desart, or rather in some greate Citty laid waste by a cruel enemy; to which was added the stench that came from some poore creatures bodies, beds, and other combustible goods. Sir Tho. Gressham's statue, tho' fallen from its nich in the Royal Exchange, remain'd intire, when all those of the Kings since the Conquest were broken to pieces; also the standard in Cornehill, and Q. Elizabeth's effigies, with some armes on Ludgate, continued with but little detriment, whilst the vast yron chaines of the Citty streetes, hinges, barrs and gates of prisons were many of them mealted and reduced to cinders by the vehement heate. Nor was I yet able to passe through any of the narrower streetes, but kept the widest; the ground and aire, smoake and fiery vapour, continu'd so intense that my haire was almost sing'd, and my feete unsufferably surbated. The bie lanes and narrower streetes were quite fill'd up with rubbish, nor could one have possibly knowne where he was, but by the ruines of some Church or Hall, that had some remarkable tower or pinnacle remaining (172).'

Leaving the City, Evelyn went to the open fields northwards where the refugees from the Fire had encamped: 'I then went towards Islington and Highgate, where one might have seene 200,000

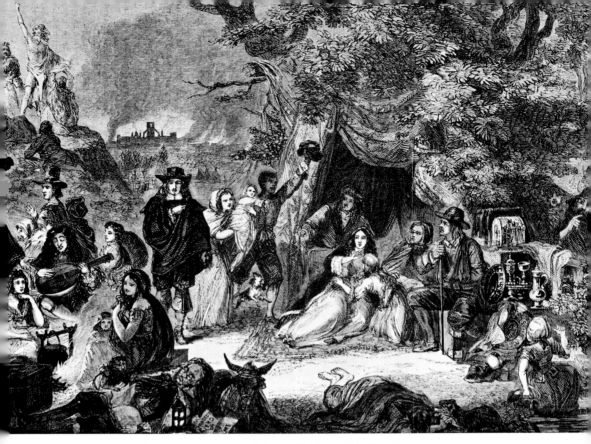

The homeless camping out in Highgate Fields outside London

people of all ranks and degrees dispers'd and lying along by their heapes of what they could save from the fire, deploring their losse, and tho' ready to perish for hunger and destitution, yet not asking one pennie for reliefe, which to me appear'd a stranger sight than any I had yet beheld. His Majesty and Council indeede tooke all imaginable care for their reliefe ... (173).'

Evelyn visits the refugees

Pepys also went out on Friday morning to view the scene of the Fire: 'Up by five o'clock, and blessed be God! find all well; and by water to Paul's Wharfe. Walked thence and saw all the towne burned, and a miserable sight of Paul's church, with all the roofs fallen, and the body of the quire fallen into St Fayth's; Paul's school also, Ludgate, and Fleet-street, my father's house and the church and a good part of the Temple the like. So to Creed's lodging near the New Exchange, and there find him laid down upon a bed, the house all unfurnished, there being fears of the fire's

Pepys inspects the ruins

101

coming to them. There borrowed a shirt of him and washed (174).'

First he had a talk with Sir William Coventry, Secretary to the Duke of York: 'To Sir W. Coventry at St James's, who lay without curtains, having removed all his goods, as the King at White Hall and every body had done and was doing. He hopes we shall have no publique distractions upon this fire, which is what every body fears, because of the talke of the French having a hand in it. And it is a proper time for discontents; but all men's minds are full of care to protect themselves and save their goods. The militia is in armes every where. Our fleetes, he tells me, have been in sight one of another, and most unhappily by fowle weather were parted, to our great losse. So home and did give orders for my house to be made clean (175).'

Getting back to normal
The rest of the day was spent in the difficult task of recovering from the effects of the Fire: 'This day our Merchants first met at Gresham College, which, by proclamation, is to be their Exchange. Strange to hear what is bid for houses all up and down here, a friend of Sir W. Rider's having £150 for what he used to let for £40 per annum. Much dispute where the Customehouse shall be; thereby the growth of the City again to be foreseen. I home late to Sir W. Pen's, who did give me a bed, but without curtains or hangings, all being down. So here I went the first time into a naked bed, only my drawers on, and did sleep pretty well; but still both sleeping and waking had a fear of fire in my heart, that I took little rest. People do all the world over cry out of the simplicity of my Lord Mayor in generall; and more particularly in this business of the fire, laying it all upon him. A proclamation is come out for markets to be kept at Leadenhall and Mile-end-greene and several other places about the towne, and Tower-hill; and all churches to be set open to receive poor people (176).'

On Saturday, he spoke with the merchants of the City: 'To Gresham College, where infinity of people, partly through novelty to see the new place and partly to find out and hear what is become one man of another. I met with many people undone, and more that have extraordinary great losses. People speaking their thoughts variously about the beginning of the fire and the rebuilding of the City (177).' Speculation ran rife and rumour ran wild throughout the metropolis.

Later Pepys enjoyed dinner and gossip with the Surveyor of the
Navy: 'Then to Sir W. Batten's and took my brother with me, and
there dined with a great company of neighbours, and much good
discourse; among others of the low spirits of some rich men in the
City in sparing any encouragement to the poor people that
wrought for the saving their houses. Among others Alderman
Starling, a very rich man without children, the fire at next door to
him in our lane, after our men had saved his house did give 2*s*. 6*d*.
among thirty of them, and did quarrel with some that would
remove the rubbish out of the way of the fire, saying that they come
to steal. Sir W. Coventry told me of another this morning in Holborne, which he shewed the King: that when it was offered to stop
the fire near his house for such a reward that came but to 2*s*. 6*d*.
a man among the neighbours he would give but 18*d*. (178).'

On Sunday, a week after the outbreak of the Fire, he heard a
sermon he did not appreciate: 'To church, and there preached
Dean Harding, but methinks a bad, poor sermon, though proper
for the time; nor eloquent in saying at this time that the City is
reduced from a large folio to a decimo-tertio (179).'

Pepys began the week after the Fire 'All the morning clearing
our cellars, and breaking in pieces all my old lumber to make room
and to prevent fire (180).'

Clarendon observed that the country people continued their
kindness towards the distressed Londoners: 'And which was more
miraculous, in our days, in all the fields about the town, which had
seemed covered with those whose habitations were burned, and
with the goods which they had saved, there was scarce a man to
be seen: all found shelter in so short a time, either in those parts
which remained of the city and in the suburbs, or in the neighbour
villages; all kind of people expressing a marvellous charity towards
those who appeared to be undone. And very many, with more
expedition than can be conceived, set up little sheds of brick and
timber upon the ruins of their own houses, where they chose rather
to inhabit than in more convenient places, though they knew they
could not long reside in those new buildings (181).'

A clergyman wrote, as he recalled the wreckage of the Fire: 'A
ruinous confused place the City was by Chimneys and Steeples
only standing in the midst of Cellars, and heaps of Rubbish; so

it was hard to know where the streets had been ... No man that seeth not such a thing, can have a right apprehension of the dreadfullness of it (182).'

Another alarm   In November 1666, the Horse Guards opposite the Banqueting Hall in Whitehall blazed up. Pepys was dining with friends at Whitehall when it started: 'And so we run up to the garret, and find it so; a horrid great fire; and by and by we saw and heard part of it being blown up with powder. The ladies begun presently to be afraid: one fell into fits. The whole town in alarum. Drums beat and trumpets, and the Horse Guards every where spread, running up and down in the street. By and by comes the news that the fire is slackened; so then we were a little cheered up again, and to supper and pretty merry. After supper, another dance or two, and then news that the fire is as great as ever, which puts us all to our wit's-end; and I mighty anxious to get home ... [but] by people coming from the fire, understood that the fire was overcome and all well, we merrily parted, and home (183).'

And for months the flames sprang to life again as cellars were opened. As late as March 1667, Pepys wrote: 'The weather is now grown warm again, after much cold; and it is observable that within these eight days I did see smoke remaining, coming out of some cellars, from the late great fire, now about six months since (184).'

A new menace   An extract from a letter, written in December 1666 by James Hickes, the Acting Postmaster, refers to the thieves and murderers who hid in the deserted cellars and vaults that autumn: 'There are many people found murdered and carried into the vaults among the ruins, as three last night as I hear, and it is supposed by hasty fellows that cry 'Do you want a light?' and carry links [torches]; and that when they catch a man single, whip into a vault with him knock him down, strip him from top to toe, blow out their links, and leave the persons for dead (185).'

A scapegoat hanged   A Frenchman, Robert Hubert, was hanged in October 1666 for starting the Fire, though it was later discovered that he was not even in England when the Fire began. This is the True Bill presented by the jury at his trial: '*London*. The jury for our Lord the King present upon their oath that Robert Hubert, late of London, labourer, not having the fear of God before his eyes, but moved

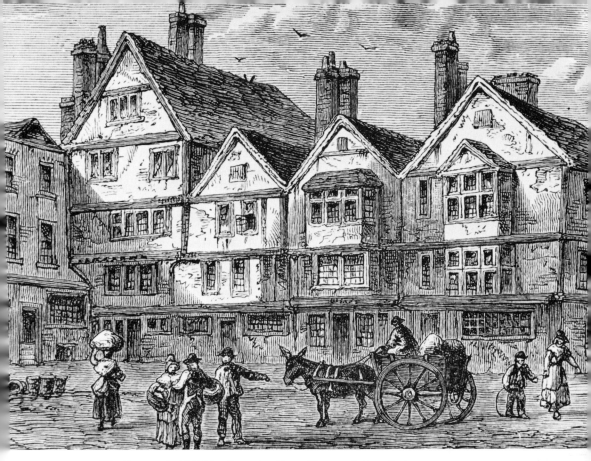

Pie Corner, Smithfield, where the Great Fire reached its limits

and led away by the instigation of the devil, on the 2nd day of
September, 18 Charles II., about the second hour of the night of
that day, with force and arms, etc., in London, to wit, in the parish
of St Margaret New Fishstreete, in the ward of Billingsgate,
London aforesaid, a fireball by the same Robert Hubert com-
pounded and made with gunpowder, brimstone and other combustible materials, and by the same Robert then and there kindled
and fired, then and there voluntarily, maliciously and feloniously
did throw into the mansion house of one Thomas Farriner the
elder, baker, set and being in Pudding-lane in the parish and ward
aforesaid; and with the fireball aforesaid by the same Robert
Hubert thus, as aforesaid, kindled and fired, and thrown into the
said mansion house, did then and there devilishly, feloniously,
voluntarily, and of his malice aforethought set on fire, burn, and

105

wholly destroy not only the said mansion house of the aforesaid Thomas Farriner, but also a great number of churches and other mansion houses and buildings of thousands of lieges and subjects of our Lord the King, set and being in the parish and ward aforesaid, and in the said city of London and the suburbs thereof, contrary to the peace of our said Lord the now King, his Crown and dignity (186).'

9 Rebuilding the City

HERE is an extract from a report by two surveyors, Jonas Moore and Ralph Gatrix, who charted the devastated area: ' "Upon the 2nd of September, 1666," they wrote, "the Fire began in London at one Farryner's house, a baker, in Pudding-lane, between the hours of one and two in the morning, and continued burning until the 6th of September following: consuming three hundred and 73 acres within the wall of the City of London, and 63 acres, three roods without the walls.

'There remains 75 acres three roods yet standing within the walls unburnt. Eighty-nine parish churches, besides chapels, burnt: eleven parishes within the walls yet standing. Houses burnt, 13,200." (187).'

Clarendon observed that, unlike the Plague, the Fire struck at the wealthiest area of London: 'The effect was very terrible; for above two parts of three of that great city were burned to ashes, and those the most rich and wealthy parts of the city, where the greatest warehouses and the best shops stood. The Royal Exchange, with all the streets about it, Lombard-street, Cheapside, Paternoster-row, St Paul's church, and almost all the other churches in the city, with the Old Bailey, Ludgate, all Paul's churchyard even to the Thames, and the greatest part of Fleet-street, all which were places the best inhabited, were all burned without one house remaining (188).'

Here are two items from a calculation of the losses suffered by London's merchants, which has been attributed to Sir Christopher Wren: 'Wine, tobacco, sugar, plums etc., of which the City was at that time very full—£1,500,000; Wares, household-stuff, monies and movable goods lost and spoilt—£2,000,000 (189).'

Extracts from the St Paul's Cathedral account book for the winter of 1666–7: 'Charges for removing the records of that Church [St Paul's at the time of the Great Fire] and securing them at Fulham; for portage, lighterage, watching etc ... £5–0–0. For boat hire twice, and portage of the records from Fulham to London, and for one burden from Dr Barwick ... £0–9–8. For printing Enquiries after some of that Furniture of the Church lost at the Fire to be posted and dispersed in several places ... £1–0–0. To the 6 Lay Vicars [Choral] For carrying the Copes and for other services in the Choir ... £2–3–4. To the Bell-ringers for feeding the Dogs that guard that Church [St Paul's] £1–6–8 (190).'

Churches and taverns
Pepys gave some figures about churches and taverns: 'It is observed, and is true that in the late fire of London, the fire burned just as many Parish Churches as there were hours from the beginning to the end of the fire; and, next, that there were just as many churches left standing as there were taverns left standing in the rest of the City that was not burned, being, I think, thirteen in all of each: which is pretty to observe (191).'

New building ideas
In a letter written in September 1666, Evelyn spoke of the new ideas which were being put forward for the rebuilding: 'The King & Parliament are infinitely zealous for the rebuilding of our ruines; & I believe it will universally be the employment of ye next spring: They are now busied with adjusting the claimes of each proprietor, that so they may dispose things for the building after the noblest model: Every body brings in his idea ... and truly there was never a more glorious phoenix upon earth, if it do at last emerge out of the cinders, and as the designe is layd, with the present fervour of ye undertakers. But these things are as yet im'ature (192).'

The plans of Wren and Evelyn
Among the plans drawn up were those by Christopher Wren (see opposite) and John Evelyn, who proposed that London should be surrounded by plantations of fragrant trees and shrubs: 'That all low grounds circumjacent to the City, especially east and south-west, be cast and contrived into square plots, or fields of twenty, thirty and forty akers or more, separated from each other by fences of double palisades or contr'-spaliars, which should enclose a plantation of an hundred and fifty or more feet deep about each field; not much unlike to what His Majesty had already begun

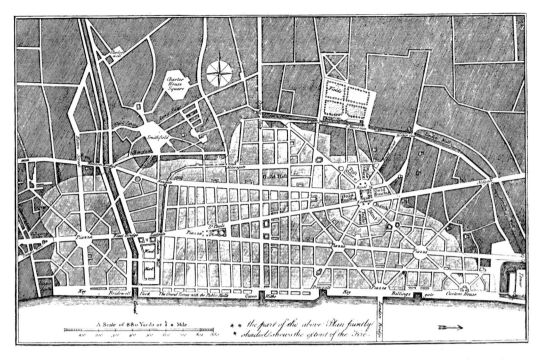

Above Wren's plan for the rebuilding of London on a regular street plan, and *below* Evelyn's plan which laid more emphasis on new parks and squares. In the end neither was adopted

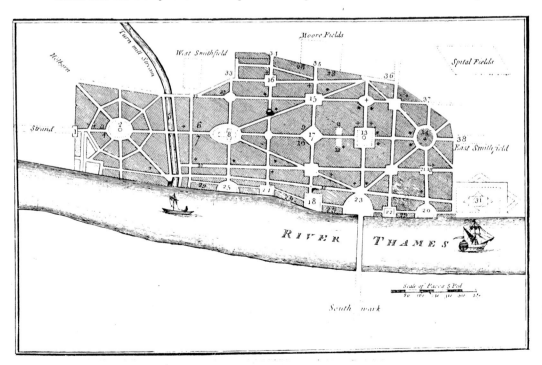

by the wall from Old Spring Garden to St James in that park; and is somewhat resembled in the new Spring Garden in Lambeth. That these palisads be elegantly planted, diligently kept and supply'd with such shrubs as yield the most fragrant and odoriferous flowers and aptest to tinge the aer upon every gentle emission at a great distance (193).'

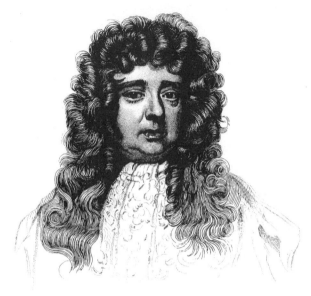

Sir William Petty

Petty's plan   Sir William Petty, the economist, estimated that London's population would be five million by 1702 and ten million by 1742. To provide for this he imagined in his plan that: 'A circle of ground of 35 miles semi-diameter will bear corn, garden stuff, fruits, hay and timber ... so that nothing of that kind need be brought above 35 miles distance from the said City; for the number of acres within the said Circle, reckoning one acre sufficient to furnish Bread and Drink of Corn for every Head, and two acres will furnish Hay for every Necessary Horse; and that the Trees which may grow in the Hedge-Rows of the Fields within the said Circle, may furnish Timber for 600 thousand Houses. That all live Cattel and great Animals can bring themselves to the said City; and that Fish can be brought from the Lands-End and Berwick as easily as now. Of coals there is no doubt; and for Water, 20s. per Family (or 600 Thousand pounds per Annum in the Whole) will serve this City, especially with the help of the New River (194).'

An extract from a letter by Henry Oldenburg, Secretary of the Royal Society, written in September 1666, tells us that: 'The re- *Planning difficulties*

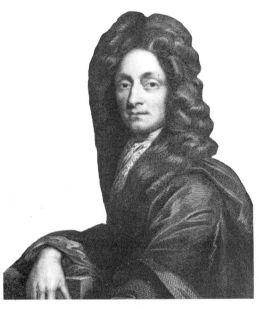

Sir Christopher Wren

building of the citty, as to the model, is still very perplext, there appearing three parties in the house of commons about it. Some are for a quite new model, according to Dr Wren's draught; some are for the old, yet to build with bricks; others for a middle way, by building a key, and enlarging some streets, but keeping the old foundations and vaults. I hear, this very day there is a meeting of some of his majesties councill, and others of the nobility, with the leading men of the citty, to conferre about this great work, and to try, whether they can bring it to some issue, before the people, that inhabited London, doe scatter into other parts. The great stresse will be, how to raise mony for carrying on the warre, and to rebuild the citty at the same time (195).'

After talking with Hugh May, the City's Solicitor, in November,

111

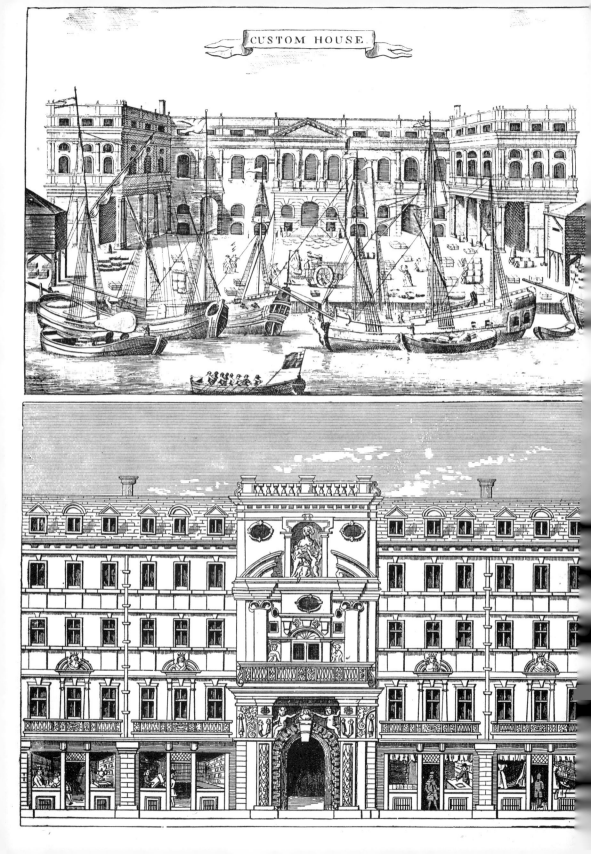

CUSTOM HOUSE.

Pepys doubted whether any of the plans would be put into effect: 'I spoke with Mr May, who tells me that the design of building the City do go on apace, and by his description it will be mighty handsome, and to the satisfaction of the people; but I pray God it come not out too late (196).'

In the end, none of the plans was adopted. The Rebuilding Act decreed that the City should be rebuilt on the old street plan and to enable it to take place as quickly as possible, it compelled the guilds to lift their restrictions on the employment of skilled craftsmen in London: 'All carpenters, bricklayers, masons, plasterers, joiners, and other artificers, workmen and labourers to be employed in the said buildings, who are not freemen of the said City [of London] shall for the space of seven years next ensuing, and for so long time after as until the said buildings shall be fully finished, have and enjoy such and the same liberty of working, and being set to work in the said building, as the freemen of the City of the same trades and professions have and ought to enjoy; Any usage or custom of the City to the contrary notwithstanding. And that such artificers as aforesaid, which for the space of seven years shall have wrought in the rebuilding of the City in their respective arts, shall from and after the said seven years have and enjoy the same liberty to work as freemen of the said City for and during their natural lives (197).' *The Rebuilding Act 1667*

Dr Nicholas Barbon, son of the Puritan 'Praise-God Barebones', was a speculative builder, who undertook a number of schemes after the Fire. One of his most successful operations was the development of the site of Essex House on the Strand. Strype's *Survey of London* said of this: 'Almost against St Clement's Church is an open passage into Essex Street or Building, being a broad clean and handsome street, especially beyond the turning into the Temple, where it crosseth Little Essex Street into Milford Lane; it consisteth of two rows of good built houses, well inhabited by gentry; at the bottom of which is a pair of stairs to go down to the waterside where watermen ply ... of late the passage into it (Essex Street) out of the great street is widened and made more convenient. Out of this Essex Street westwards is a small street or passage for carts called Little Essex Street, which leadeth to Milford Lane (198).' *A speculative builder*

Facing page: top The new Custom House built two years after the Great Fire had destroyed the old one, and *below* the Mercers' Chapel as rebuilt after the Fire
Overleaf View of London and the Thames after the Great Fire

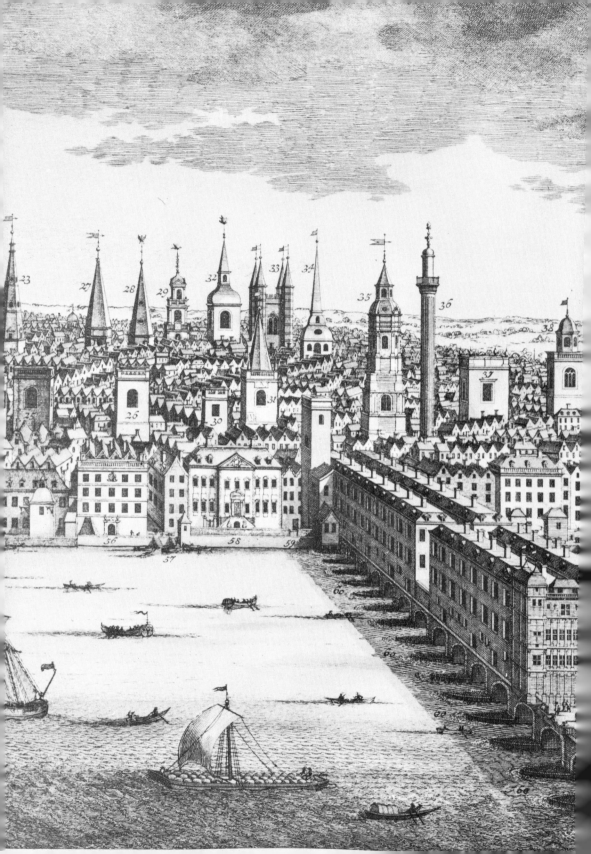

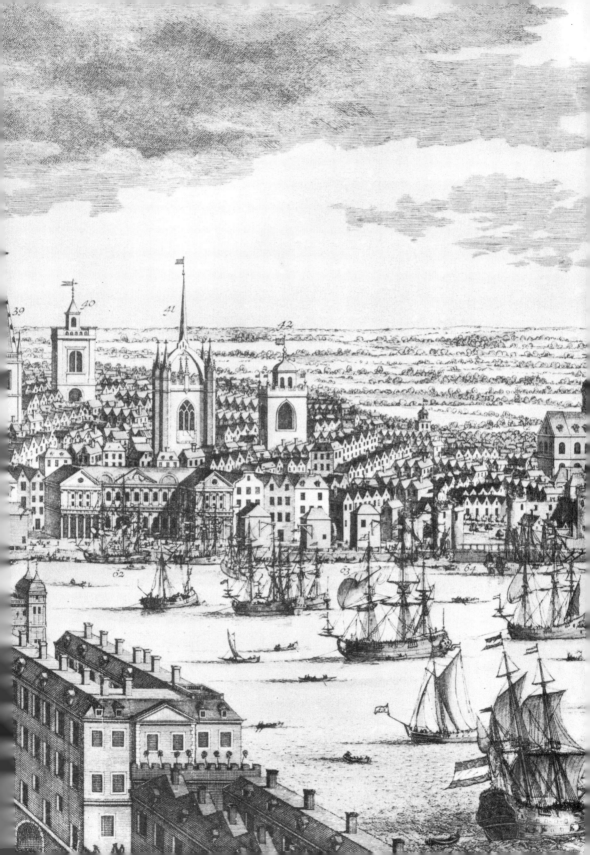

Narcissus Luttrell told in his diary of an unsuccessful attempt by the lawyers of Gray's Inn in June 1684 to stop Barbon building Red Lion Square: 'Dr Barebone, the great builder, having some time since bought the Red Lyon Fields near Gray's Inn Walks to build on, and having for that purpose employed several workmen to goe on with the same, the Gentlemen of Gray's Inn took notice of it, and thinking it an injury to them, went with a considerable body of 100 persons; upon which the workmen assaulted the gentlemen and threw bricks at them again; so a sharp engagement ensued, but the gentlemen routed them at the last and brought away one or two of the workmen to Graie's Inn; in this skirmish one or two of the gentlemen and servants of the House were hurt, and several of the workmen (199).'

The Monument   The Monument, erected close to where the Fire started, had from 1681 to 1830 this inscription: 'This pillar was set up in perpetual remembrance of that most dreadful burning of this Protestant city, begun and carried on by ye treachery & malice of ye Popish faction in ye year of our Lord 1665, in order for carrying on their horrid plott for extirpating the Protestant and old English liberty, and introducing Popery and slavery (200).'

Where the fire   Set into the wall of the house built on the site of the baker's
started   house in Pudding Lane, where the Fire started, was a stone (now in the Guildhall Museum) bearing this inscription: 'Here by ye permission of Heaven Hell broke loose upon this Protestant City from the Malicious Hearts of Barbarous Papists, by ye hand of their agent Hubert, who Confessed, and on ye Ruines of this Place declared the fact, for which he was hanged, (vizt.) that here began that Dredfull Fire, which is described and perpetuated on and by the neighbouring Pillar.

Erected Anno 168[1, i]n the Majoraltie of Sr Patience Ward Kt. (201).'

The new St   In the autumn of 1694 Evelyn visited the rising new cathedral:
Paul's   'I went to St Paul's to see the choir now finished as to the stone work, and the scaffolds struck both without and within, in that part. Some exception might perhaps be taken as to the placing columns on pilasters at the eastern tribunal. As to the rest it is a piece of architecture without reproach (202).'

116   To Clarendon the speedy restoration of the City was amazing:

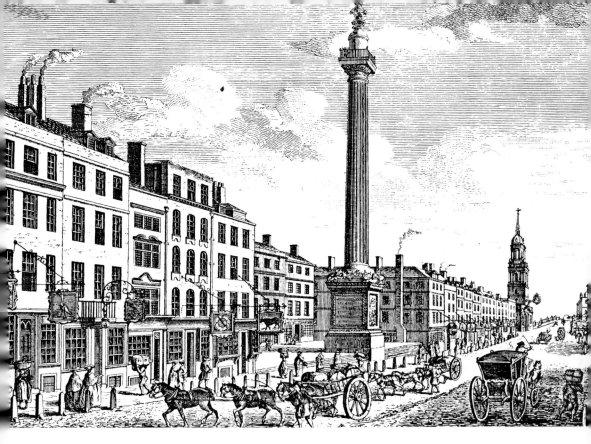

A view of the Monument to the Great Fire

'The so sudden repair of those formidable ruins, and the giving so great beauty to all deformity, (a beauty and a lustre that city had never before been acquainted with,) is little less wonderful than the fire that consumed it (203).'

By 1672, indeed, the greater part of the destroyed areas had been *A better city* rebuilt, and London was a healthier and finer town. Dr Woodward, a lecturer at Gresham College, wrote to Wren to sum up the result: 'The Fire however disastrous it might be to the then inhabitants, had prov'd infinitely beneficial to their Posterity; conducing vastly to the Improvement and Increase, as well of the Riches and Opu-

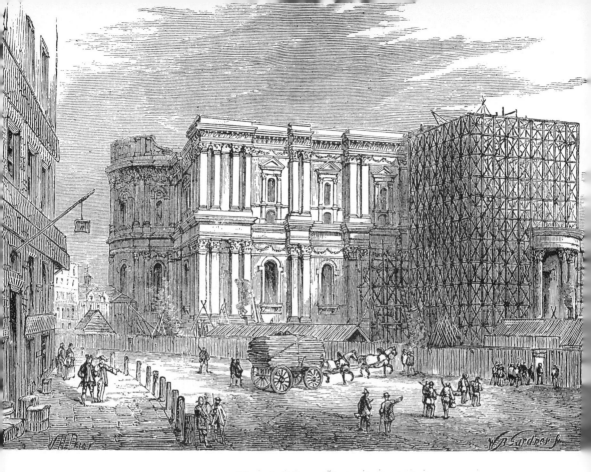

The rebuilding of St Paul's Cathedral

lency, as of the Splendor of this City. Then, which I and every
Body must observe with great Satisfaction, by means of the In-
largements of the Streets; of the great Plenty of good Water,
convey'd to all Parts; of the common Sewers, and other like Con-
trivances, such Provision is made for a free Access and Passage
of the Air, for Sweetness, for Cleanness, and for Salubrity, that
it is not only the finest, but the most healthy City in the World
(204).'

Picture Credits

Sources

(1) Iona & Peter Opie, *Oxford Dictionary of Nursery Rhymes* (1951), pp. 364–5.
(2) James Leasor, *The Plague and the Fire* (Pan Books, 1962), p. 26.
(3) *Ibid*, p. 19.
(4) R. J. Mitchell & M. D. R. Leys, *A History of London Life* (Penguin Books, 1963), p. 175.
(5) W. G. Bell, *The Great Plague in London* (Bodley Head, 1924), p. 144.
(6) Mitchell & Leys, *op. cit.*, 123.
(7) Leasor, *op. cit.*, p. 44.
(8) *Ibid*, p. 45.
(9) *Ibid*, p. 44.
(10) Daniel Defoe, *A Journal of the Plague Year* (Everyman Edition, 1948), pp. 21–3.
(11) Bell, *op. cit.*, p. 3.
(12) *Selections from Clarendon*, ed. G. Huehns (World's Classics, 1955), p. 410.
(13) *The Verneys of Claydon*, ed. Sir Harry Verney (Pergamon, 1968), p. 159.
(14) Bell, *op. cit.*, p. 28.
(15) Leasor, *op. cit.*, p. 28.
(16) *Ibid*, p. 27.
(17) Defoe, *op. cit.*, p. 34.
(18) *Ibid*, p. 37.
(19) *Clarendon*, p. 411.
(20) *Ibid*, p. 411.
(21) *Ibid*, pp. 411–12.
(22) *Ibid*, p. 412.

(23)   *Ibid*, p. 412.
(24)   *Ibid*, p. 412.
(25)   Samuel Pepys, *Diary*, 30 April 1665.
(26)   Leasor, *op. cit.*, p. 34.
(27)   Defoe, *op. cit.*, p. 37.
(28)   *The Verneys*, p. 159.
(29)   Leasor, *op. cit.*, p. 53.
(30)   *Clarendon*, pp. 412–13.
(31)   Pepys, 7 June 1665.
(32)   *Ibid*, 17 June 1665.
(33)   Defoe, *op. cit.*,
(34)   Pepys, 21 June 1665.
(35)   Pepys, 22 June 1665.
(36)   Bell, *op. cit.*, p. 52.
(37)   Defoe, *op. cit.*, p. 172.
(38)   *Ibid*, p. 121.
(39)   Leasor, *op. cit.*, p. 145.
(40)   *Ibid*, p. 145.
(41)   Richard Baxter, *Autobiography* (Everyman Edition, 1931), p. 195.
(42)   Defoe, *op. cit.*, pp. 88–9.
(43)   *Ibid*, pp. 118–19.
(44)   *Ibid*, p. 19.
(45)   Pepys, 28 August 1665.
(46)   Bell, *op. cit.*, pp. 230–1.
(47)   *Ibid*, p. 92.
(48)   Defoe, *op. cit.*, pp. 59–60.
(49)   Bell, *op. cit.*, p. 107.
(50)   *Ibid*, p. 110.
(51)   *Ibid*, pp. 333–4.
(52)   *Ibid*, pp. 334–5.
(53)   Leasor, *op. cit.*, p. 166.
(54)   Defoe, *op cit.*, p. 67.
(55)   *Ibid*, pp. 102–3.
(56)   Leasor, *op. cit.*, p. 68.
(57)   Bell, *op. cit.*, pp. 80–1.
(58)   John Evelyn, *Diary*, 16 July, 8 & 15 August 1665.
(59)   *Ibid*, 2 August 1665.

(60) Pepys, 15 August 1665.
(61) Leasor, *op. cit.*, pp. 57–8.
(62) *Ibid*, p. 59.
(63) *Ibid*, p. 59.
(64) *Ibid*, p. 69.
(65) Pepys, 4 September 1665.
(66) Bell, *op. cit.*, p. 133.
(67) Leasor, *op. cit.*, p. 149.
(68) *Ibid*, p. 126.
(69) *Ibid*, p. 127.
(70) *Ibid*, p. 127.
(71) Pepys, 31 August 1665.
(72) *Ibid*, 3 September 1665.
(73) *Ibid*, 6 September 1665.
(74) Defoe, *op. cit.*, p. 249.
(75) Pepys, 3 September 1665.
(76) *Ibid*, 3 September 1665.
(77) *Ibid*, 4 September 1665.
(78) *Ibid*, 8 January 1666.
(79) *Ibid*, 20 September 1665.
(80) Evelyn, 11 October 1665.
(81) Pepys, 24 November 1665.
(82) *Clarendon*, p. 413.
(83) Pepys, 30 November 1665.
(84) Defoe, *op. cit.*, p. 257.
(85) Bell, *op. cit.*, p. 285.
(86) Defoe, *op. cit.*, p. 274.
(87) Evelyn, 31 December 1665.
(88) Pepys, 31 December 1665.
(89) Pepys, 5 January 1666.
(90) Defoe, *op. cit.*, p. 264.
(91) Pepys, 4 February 1666.
(92) Baxter, *op. cit.*, p. 195.
(93) Leasor, *op. cit.*, p. 196.
(94) Bell, *op. cit.*, p. 331.
(95) J. E. N. Hearsey, *Bridge, Church and Palace* (Murray, 1961), p. 55.
(96) Mitchell & Leys, *op. cit.*, p. 173.

(97) *Clarendon*, p. 413.
(98) G. Burnet, *History of His Own Times* (Everyman Edition, 1932), p. 80.
(99) Pepys, 2 September 1666.
(100) *Ibid*, 2 September 1666.
(101) *Ibid*, 2 September 1666.
(102) W. G. Bell, *The Great Fire of London* (Bodley Head, 1920), p. 32.
(103) Pepys, 2 September 1666.
(104) *Ibid*, 2 September 1666.
(105) *Ibid*, 2 September 1666.
(106) *Ibid*, 2 September 1666.
(107) Leasor, *op. cit.*, p. 220.
(108) *Clarendon*, p. 414.
(109) *Ibid*, p. 414.
(110) *The Verneys*, p. 167.
(111) Bell, *op. cit.*, p. 33.
(112) Pepys, 2 September 1666.
(113) *Ibid*, 2 September 1666.
(114) *Ibid*, 2 September 1666.
(115) *Clarendon*, p. 416.
(116) Evelyn, 3 September 1666.
(117) Pepys, 3 September 1666.
(118) *Ibid*, 3 September 1666.
(119) *The Verneys*, p. 165.
(120) Pepys, 3 September 1666.
(121) *Clarendon*, p. 417.
(122) Evelyn, 3 September 1666.
(123) Baxter, *op. cit.*, p. 198.
(124) *Clarendon*, p. 417.
(125) *Ibid*, p. 417.
(126) Leasor, *op. cit.*, p. 231.
(127) *Ibid*, p. 231.
(128) Evelyn, 3 September 1666.
(129) Leasor, *op. cit.*, p. 230.
(130) Evelyn, 3 September 1666.
(131) *Ibid*, 3 September 1666.
(132) *Ibid*, 3 September 1666.

(133) Pepys, 4 September 1666.
(134) Bell, *op. cit.*, p. 94.
(135) Evelyn, 4 September 1666.
(136) *Ibid*, 4 September 1666.
(137) Pepys, 4 September 1666.
(138) Evelyn, 4 September 1666.
(139) Pepys, 4 September 1666.
(140) Evelyn, 4 September 1666.
(141) Pepys, 4 September 1666.
(142) Evelyn, 4 September 1666.
(143) *Clarendon*, p. 418.
(144) *Ibid*, p. 418.
(145) *Ibid*, p. 419.
(146) Leasor, *op. cit.*, pp. 237–8.
(147) Bell, *op. cit.*, p. 134.
(148) J. E. N. Hearsey, *London and the Great Fire* (Murray 1965), pp. 154–5.
(149) Leasor, *op. cit.*, p. 243.
(150) Pepys, 5 September 1666.
(151) *Ibid*, 5 September 1666.
(152) *Ibid*, 5 September 1666.
(153) *Ibid*, 4 September 1666.
(154) *Ibid*, 4 September 1666.
(155) *Ibid*, 4 September 1666.
(156) Evelyn, 4 September 1666.
(157) Leasor, *op. cit.*, p. 225.
(158) Hearsey, *op. cit.*, 145.
(159) *Ibid*, p. 165.
(160) Bell, *op. cit.*, p. 137.
(161) *Ibid*, p. 137.
(162) *Ibid*, p. 137.
(163) Hearsey, *op. cit.*, pp. 158–9.
(164) Pepys, 6 September 1666.
(165) *Ibid*, 6 September 1666.
(166) *Ibid*, 6 September 1666.
(167) Hearsey, *op. cit.*, p. 159.
(168) Pepys, 4 October 1666.
(169) Evelyn, 7 September 1666.

(170) *Ibid*, 7 September 1666.
(171) *Ibid*, 7 September 1666.
(172) *Ibid*, 7 September 1666.
(173) *Ibid*, 7 September 1666.
(174) Pepys, 7 September 1666.
(175) *Ibid*, 7 September 1666.
(176) *Ibid*, 7 September 1666.
(177) *Ibid*, 8 September 1666.
(178) *Ibid*, 8 September 1666.
(179) *Ibid*, 9 September 1666.
(180) *Ibid*, 10 September 1666.
(181) *Clarendon*, pp. 419–20.
(182) Leasor, *op. cit.*, p. 253.
(183) Pepys, 9 November 1666.
(184) *Ibid*, 16 March 1667.
(185) Bell, *op. cit.*, p. 191.
(186) *Ibid*, p. 354.
(187) Leasor, *op. cit.*, pp. 251–2.
(188) *Clarendon*, p. 421.
(189) Leasor, *op. cit.*, p. 252.
(190) W. R. Matthews & W. R. Atkins (edd.), *A History of St Paul's Cathedral* (Phoenix, 1957), pp. 193–4.
(191) Pepys, 10 November 1666.
(192) T. F. Reddaway, *The Rebuilding of London* (Cape, 1940), p. 54.
(193) N. G. Brett-James, *The Growth of Stuart London* (Allen & Unwin, 1935), p. 313.
(194) *Ibid*, p. 322.
(195) Reddaway, *op. cit.*, p. 55.
(196) Pepys, 25 November 1666.
(197) Bell, *op. cit.*, p. 254.
(198) Reddaway, *op. cit.*, p. 327.
(199) Brett-James, *op. cit.*, p. 330.
(200) Eric de Maré, *London's Riverside* (Reinhardt, 1958), p. 110.
(201) Bell, *op. cit.*, p. 298.
(202) Evelyn, 5 October 1694.
(203) *Clarendon*, p. 243.
(204) Reddaway, *op. cit.*, p. 300.

Index